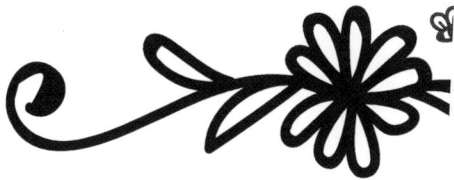

FOOD JOURNAL

By Your Side, Every Day.

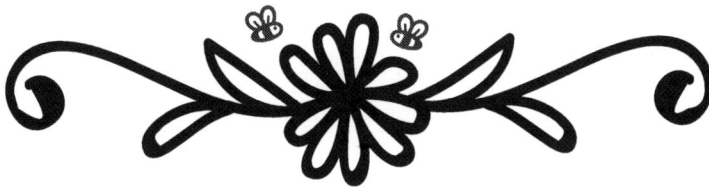

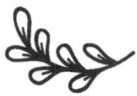

Welcome

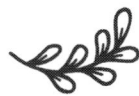

Welcome dear friend! If you are reading these lines you probably can't wait to start fill in your diary, but please allow me to take five minutes of your time to tell you why I wanted to publish it.

I did it for two reasons: to help you improve your physical fitness and help you achieve a state of general well-being that will allow you to build the Best Version of Yourself. I said "help you" because this is a mission that we will have to accomplish together, I will guide you, but you will have to do the most important part.

But don't worry, the good news is you've already start-ed doing it!

By opening it **you have already taken the First Step**, the fundamental one, the step that will lead you to reach any goal you want. You have decided to START moving towards your goal.

During these 90 days I will be here to motivate you, be-cause you probably have also started something with the best intentions, but at the end of the day, for one reason or another, you have not been able to complete it.

When the final goal is too big, or too far away, sooner or later you lose sight of it and the motivation to reach it may decrease.

If we break down this goal into many smaller goals, we will achieve the result by being able to reach them one

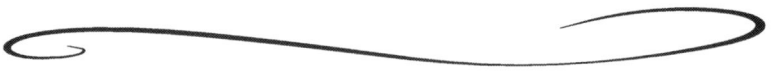

after the other, and the gratification for having succeed-ed will be our drive to move forward, increasingly moti-vated and increasingly satisfied.

This is what I call the baby steps technique: one step at a time, one day at a time, one small goal at a time, you get to the end of the road realizing what we promised.

Small steps require a minimum effort, we can do them easily, the most important thing to do is not to make up excuses to give up. During these 90 days, a bad day will probably make it harder for us to do our part, but we have to insist.

Our mind seems tailored to find excuses: work, lack of time, family, etc. They all seem like great reasons to stop, but we have to be good at not being fooled by our own brains and not sabotaging ourselves.

If the goal is small and achievable, there can be no obsta-cle that can stop us!

Give yourself a little gift at the end of the week if you were able to achieve the small step that was proposed to you.

This may seem strange to you, but our brain will begin to associate good behavior with a reward, motivated by receiving the reward it will stop making us find excuses not to commit ourselves.

You can feed this unconscious behavior if you spend 2 minutes every day thinking about your reward: try it in the morning and you will see that it will help you be more concentrated throughout the day.

Years of experience in the field of Good Nutrition have taught me that:
if we introduce good habits, we will manage without too much effort to improve our lifestyle and reach a state of general well-being and perfect shape.

Now I will give you the formula (which is not secret) to achieve the goals we have set ourselves:

AWARENESS + ACTION + MOTIVATION = SUCCESS

Awareness:
The diary will allow you to write down your eating habits, and will also allow you to observe and gain awareness about them. By rereading what you have written, you will be able to understand if you are doing something wrong in the right direction and you can concentrate on trying to improve that single little behavior.
If, on the other hand, by rereading what you have written, you realize that you have made improvements, this will give you additional motivation that will help you improve more and more.

Action:
Every week I will propose to you a small step to take to introduce changes in your life.
Attempt to do your best during the week.

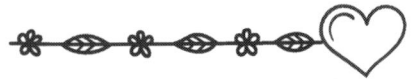

If one day you weren't able to follow the advice of the week, do not get demotivated, nothing bad happened because the next day you can immediately try again.
Please, continue to act even when you want to give up and you will change these behaviors into habits that you will never be able to give up after a while.

Motivation:
At the end of each week we will perform a check, you will have to re-read everything you have written and compile a very short summary to evaluate the improvements you have made.
Don't worry, it will take less than 5 minutes.
Just check what you wrote in the previous 7 days to find out if you were able to follow the advice of the week or to change one of the old habits by replacing it with a more suitable one to achieve your goal.

Dr. Simona Meloni.

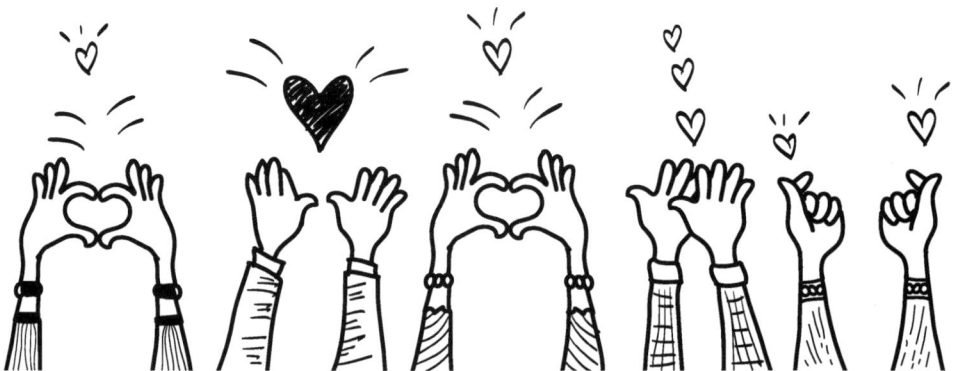

YOUR "WHYS"

Before moving on, let's stop for a moment and write down below the 3 reasons why you want to reach your goal: be as specific as you can.
The more precise the reason why you want to succeed is, the stronger the desire to succeed will be in you.
Every time you feel you have lost your motivation, reread your reasons. This way you will always have in mind WHY you want to reach them and this will give you fresh energy and a new push going forward.

I want to improve my nutrition and my lifestyle because:

....

....

....

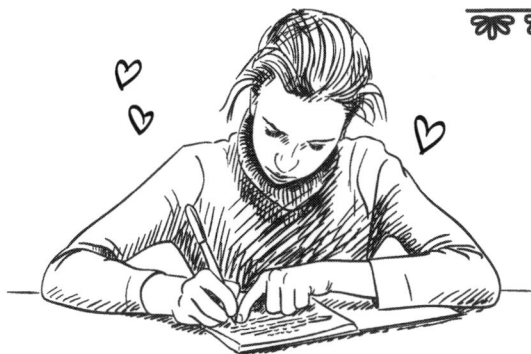

Ready for a Fresh Start?

Your measurements:

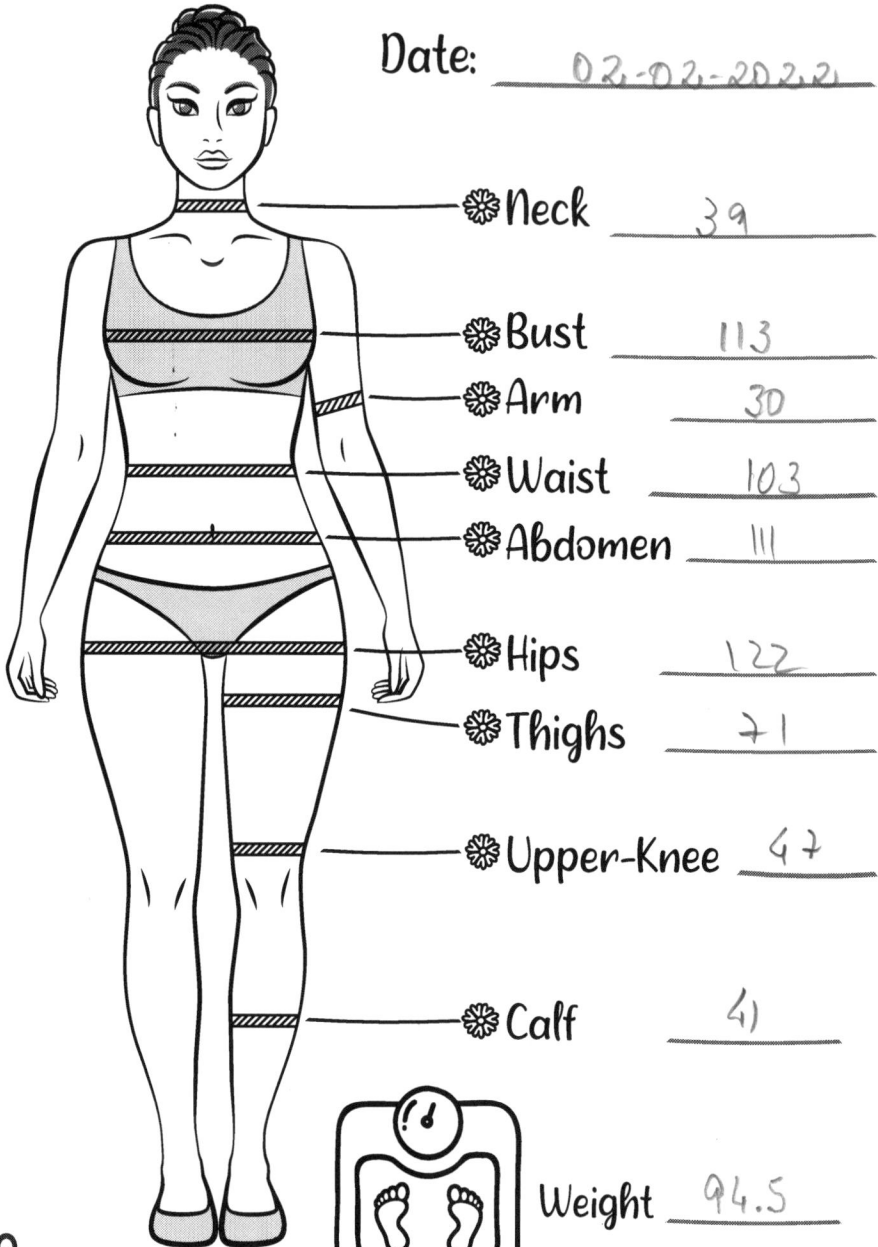

Date: _02-02-2022_

❀ Neck ___39___

❀ Bust ___113___

❀ Arm ___30___

❀ Waist ___103___

❀ Abdomen ___111___

❀ Hips ___122___

❀ Thighs ___71___

❀ Upper-Knee ___47___

❀ Calf ___41___

Weight ___94.5___

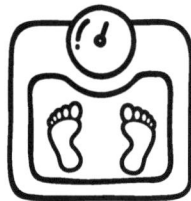
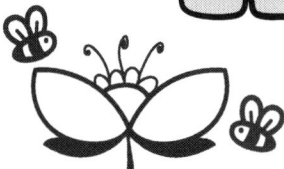
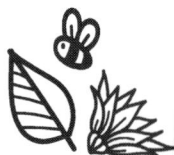

90 times the best version of yourself

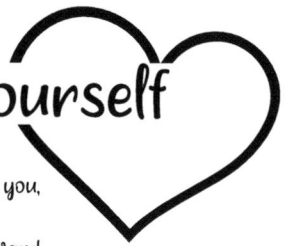

During these 90 days mark a nice "X" on the day you are filling in in the diary.
At the end of the week, if you have followed the advice that the diary has given you,
mark a nice "X" on the star!
Seeing this sheet filling up with "X's" will give you a stronger motivation to move forward
towards your goal.

First Month

Week 1   ① ② ③ ④ ⑤ ⑥ ⑦ ☆

Week 2   ⑧ ⑨ ⑩ ⑪ ⑫ ⑬ ⑭ ☆

Week 3   ⑮ ⑯ ⑰ ⑱ ⑲ ⑳ ㉑ ☆

Week 4   ㉒ ㉓ ㉔ ㉕ ㉖ ㉗ ㉘ ☆

4 WEEKS
TO ACQUIRE
NEW HABITS

Second Month

Week 5   ㉙ ㉚ ㉛ ㉜ ㉝ ㉞ ㉟ ☆

Week 6   ㊱ ㊲ ㊳ ㊴ ㊵ ㊶ ㊷ ☆

Week 7   ㊸ ㊹ ㊺ ㊻ ㊼ ㊽ ㊾ ☆

Week 8   ㊿ 51 52 53 54 55 56 ☆

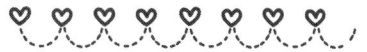

8 WEEKS
TO
START LIKING IT

Third Month

Week 9   57 58 59 60 61 62 63 ☆

Week 10   64 65 66 67 68 69 70 ☆

Week 11   71 72 73 74 75 76 77 ☆

Week 12   78 79 80 81 82 83 84 ☆

Week 13   85 86 87 88 89 90 ◎

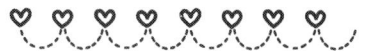

13 WEEKS
TO
CELEBRATE
YOUR
SUCCESSES

Week 1

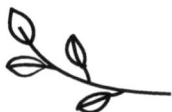
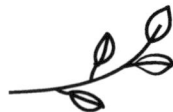

Welcome to Your First Week of this Diary!

Many people associate the word diet with a time of depriving oneself of food to lose weight, however this is not its true meaning. Did you know that the true meaning of the word diet is "Lifestyle"?

In these weeks I will ask you to take 13 small steps that will help you build a healthy lifestyle and will ensure that you no longer have to "feel you're on a diet".

You will lose weight and you will feel better from a physical and mental point of view, but above all you will learn how to manage to maintain your ideal shape over time without too many sacrifices.

This week's task is a little different from the next ones, which will be more related with how to eat, but it is just as important, indeed perhaps the most important. It's used to make you familiar with Your Diary and to change your mentality about yourself and about your diet.

Small Step of the Week:

EVERYDAY FOR 7 DAYS:

- FILL IN THE DIARY PAGE BY WRITING DOWN EVERYTHING YOU ATE (YES, EVEN IF YOU ONLY TASTED IT)
- TRY TO UNDERSTAND IF THERE HAVE BEEN ANY THINGS YOU THINK HAVE NOT GONE SO WELL
- REPEAT THESE SENTENCES TO YOURSELF:
    * I AM NOT ON A DIET: I AM IMPROVING MY LIFESTYLE.
    * I DON'T HAVE TO FEEL GUILTY IF I'M NOT IN PERFECT SHAPE: I CAN CHANGE THINGS FOR THE BETTER.
    * I DON'T HAVE TO COMPARE MYSELF TO ANYONE ELSE: MY ONLY FOCUS IS IMPROVING MYSELF.

GIVE IT A SHOT!

Day ①   Date ___ / ___ / ___

Breakfast

Lunch

Dinner

Snack 1

Snack 2

Water ____

Sleep

KCal

What time did you eat? Write B for Breakfast, S1 for Snack 1, S2 for Snack 2, L for Lunch, D for Dinner

| 5 | 6 | 7 | 8 | 9 | 10 | 11 | 12 | 13 | 14 | 15 | 16 | 17 | 18 | 19 | 20 | 21 | 22 | 23 | 24+ |

Physical Activities   Minutes / Laps / Sets / ...

- ☐ Fast Walking
- ☐ Running
- ☐ Aerobics / Zumba
- ☐ Yoga / Pilates
- ☐
- ☐

Today's Notes

Drugs & Supplements

Bad Habits

MOOD

😟 😐 😊

The journey of a thousand miles begins with one step. (Lao-Tzu)

Day ②

Date ___ / ___ / ___

Breakfast	Lunch	Dinner

Snack 1

Snack 2

🥛 Water _____

⏰ Sleep _____

🍽 KCal _____

What time did you eat? Write B for Breakfast, S1 for Snack 1, S2 for Snack 2, L for Lunch, D for Dinner

5 6 7 8 9 10 11 12 13 14 15 16 17 18 19 20 21 22 23 24+

💓 Physical Activities Minutes / Laps / Sets / ...

- ☐ Fast Walking
- ☐ Running
- ☐ Aerobics / Zumba
- ☐ Yoga / Pilates
- ☐
- ☐

🍃 Today's Notes

💊 Drugs & Supplements

🚯 Bad Habits

MOOD

😕 😐 😊

Aim for the moon. If you miss it, you will land among the stars. (Asian proverb)

Day ③

Date ___/___/___

Breakfast

_____
_____
_____
_____
_____
_____

Lunch

_____
_____
_____
_____
_____
_____

Dinner

_____
_____
_____
_____
_____
_____

Snack 1

_____
_____
_____

Snack 2

_____
_____
_____

Water _____

Sleep _____

KCal _____

What time did you eat? Write B for Breakfast, S1 for Snack 1, S2 for Snack 2, L for Lunch, D for Dinner

5	6	7	8	9	10	11	12	13	14	15	16	17	18	19	20	21	22	23	24+

♥ Physical Activities Minutes / Laps / Sets / ...

- ☐ Fast Walking _____
- ☐ Running _____
- ☐ Aerobics / Zumba _____
- ☐ Yoga / Pilates _____
- ☐ _____
- ☐ _____

Drugs & Supplements

_____
_____
_____

🚭 Bad Habits

🍃 Today's Notes

_____
_____
_____

MOOD

😞 😐 😊

Do what your heart tells you to: sing, dance, laugh and live every day of your life to the fullest.

Day ④

Date ____ / ____ / ____

Breakfast

Lunch

Dinner

Snack 1

Snack 2

Water

Sleep

KCal

What time did you eat? Write B for Breakfast, S1 for Snack 1, S2 for Snack 2, L for Lunch, D for Dinner

5 6 7 8 9 10 11 12 13 14 15 16 17 18 19 20 21 22 23 24+

Physical Activities Minutes / Laps / Sets / ...

☐ Fast Walking

☐ Running

☐ Aerobics / Zumba

☐ Yoga / Pilates

☐

☐

Today's Notes

Drugs & Supplements

Bad Habits

MOOD

Be always like the sea, than breaking up against cliffs it finds always the force to try again.
(Jim Morrison)

Day ⑤

Date ___ / ___ / ___

Breakfast

Lunch

Dinner

Snack 1

Snack 2

Water ___

Sleep ___

KCal ___

5	6	7	8	9	10	11	12	13	14	15	16	17	18	19	20	21	22	23	24+

Physical Activities Minutes / Laps / Sets / ...

☐ Fast Walking

☐ Running

☐ Aerobics / Zumba

☐ Yoga / Pilates

☐

☐

Today's Notes

Drugs & Supplements

Bad Habits

MOOD

Change your ways and your problems will solve themselves. (Anon.)

Day 6

Date ___ / ___ / ___

Breakfast

Lunch

Dinner

Snack 1

Snack 2

Water ___

Sleep ___

KCal ___

What time did you eat? Write B for Breakfast, S1 for Snack 1, S2 for Snack 2, L for Lunch, D for Dinner

5   6   7   8   9   10   11   12   13   14   15   16   17   18   19   20   21   22   23   24+

♥ Physical Activities Minutes / Laps / Sets / ...

- ☐ Fast Walking
- ☐ Running
- ☐ Aerobics / Zumba
- ☐ Yoga / Pilates
- ☐
- ☐

🌿 Today's Notes

Drugs & Supplements

Bad Habits

MOOD

😟   😐   😊

Day 7

Date _____ / _____ / _____

Breakfast

_____
_____
_____
_____
_____
_____

Lunch

_____
_____
_____
_____
_____
_____

Dinner

_____
_____
_____
_____
_____
_____

Snack 1

_____
_____
_____

Snack 2

_____
_____
_____

Water _____

Sleep _____

KCal _____

What time did you eat? Write B for Breakfast, S1 for Snack 1, S2 for Snack 2, L for Lunch, D for Dinner

5   6   7   8   9   10   11   12   13   14   15   16   17   18   19   20   21   22   23   24+

Physical Activities Minutes / Laps / Sets / ...

- ☐ Fast Walking
- ☐ Running
- ☐ Aerobics / Zumba
- ☐ Yoga / Pilates
- ☐
- ☐

Today's Notes

_____
_____

Drugs & Supplements

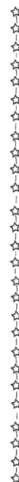

_____
_____
_____
_____

Bad Habits

MOOD

☹ 😐 🙂

If you want something you've never had,
you must be willing to do something you've never done. (T. Jefferson)

First Week Check Point:

Review what you wrote this week and answer the questions:

1) Did you fill in your diary every day?

2) Have you tried to understand if there is any mistake in your diet?

3) Have you repeated every day the 3 phrases about the right mindset?

If you answered YES to the 3 questions, you have reached this week's goal and you can mark a nice "X" on the star of Week 1. If you didn't make it, don't worry, try to understand what prevented you from doing it and we'll try again next week.

Now, if you like, you can write down your current weight, but remember not to worry too much if it's still not what you want. We will get there slowly and learn not to make it go up again.

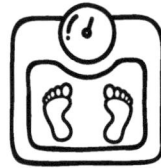

Weight
_____

Before moving on to the next tip, I want to ask you a few more questions about the week that just passed, it will help us to better evaluate your habits. In a few weeks you can come back to this page to compare the answers you have given and see how much you have improved.

In the last week ...

1) How many times have you had a snack between breakfast and lunch?

2) How many times have you had a snack between lunch and dinner?

3) How many times did you eat after dinner, before going to sleep?

4) How many times have you eaten pasta or bread?

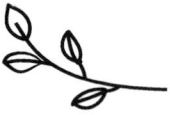

WEEK 2

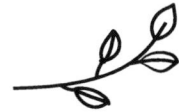

This week we will find out why, sometimes, eating more often helps us lose weight and feel better at the same time.
An excellent habit that we can introduce with little effort is to have a light snack between breakfast and lunch and another between lunch and dinner.
This will allow our body to always have all the nutrients it needs to provide us with energy and to make us feel good and in a good mood.

During this week try to divide what you eat into 5 meals and avoid "nibbling" outside these:

1. BREAKFAST
2. SNACK 1
3. LUNCH
4. SNACK 2
5. DINNER

By doing this we will never get too hungry for lunch and dinner.

Small Step of the Week:

CHOOSE 3 DAYS AND IN THESE:
- ORGANIZE YOURSELF TO HAVE 5 MEALS
- DO NOT SKIP ANY OF THESE 5 MEALS
- DO NOT EAT ANYTHING EXCEPT THESE 5 MEALS

GIVE IT A TRY!

If you are not used to have a snack, you will be surprised by how snacks they can change your day for the better, especially if you use them to eat healthy and nutritious food. Try to eat seasonal fruit, you will immediately realize how you will be able to be more focused, more energetic and in a good mood throughout the day.
Finally, remember that the snack is used to stop hunger, so it must not be too abundant. If the fruit alone is not enough to satiate you, you can also try adding some vegetables to "nibble" such as carrots or celery. ❤

Day 8

Date ___/___/___

Breakfast

_____
_____
_____
_____
_____
_____
_____
_____

Lunch

_____
_____
_____
_____
_____
_____
_____
_____

Dinner

_____
_____
_____
_____
_____
_____
_____
_____

Snack 1

_____
_____
_____
_____

Snack 2

_____
_____
_____
_____

Water _____

Sleep _____

KCal _____

What time did you eat? Write B for Breakfast, S1 for Snack 1, S2 for Snack 2, L for Lunch, D for Dinner

5	6	7	8	9	10	11	12	13	14	15	16	17	18	19	20	21	22	23	24+

Physical Activities Minutes / Laps / Sets / ...

- [ ] Fast Walking _____
- [ ] Running _____
- [ ] Aerobics / Zumba _____
- [ ] Yoga / Pilates _____
- [ ] _____
- [ ] _____

Drugs & Supplements

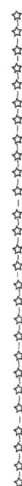

_____
_____
_____

Bad Habits

Today's Notes

_____
_____
_____

MOOD

Failure is not fatal. It is the courage to continue that counts. (W. Churchill)

Day ⑨

Date ____ / ____ / ____

Breakfast

_____
_____
_____
_____
_____
_____

Lunch

_____
_____
_____
_____
_____
_____

Dinner

_____
_____
_____
_____
_____
_____

Snack 1

_____
_____
_____

Snack 2

_____
_____
_____

Water _____

Sleep _____

KCal _____

What time did you eat? Write B for Breakfast, S1 for Snack 1, S2 for Snack 2, L for Lunch, D for Dinner

5	6	7	8	9	10	11	12	13	14	15	16	17	18	19	20	21	22	23	24+

Physical Activities Minutes / Laps / Sets / ...

☐ Fast Walking ....
☐ Running ....
☐ Aerobics / Zumba ....
☐ Yoga / Pilates ....
☐ ....
☐ ....

Today's Notes

_____

Drugs & Supplements

_____
_____
_____

Bad Habits

MOOD

😞 😐 😊

You don't have to see the whole staircase, just take the first step. (Martin Luther King)

Day 10

Date ___ / ___ / ___

Breakfast

_____
_____
_____
_____
_____
_____
_____

Lunch

_____
_____
_____
_____
_____
_____
_____

Dinner

_____
_____
_____
_____
_____
_____
_____

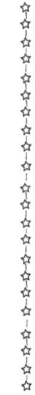

Snack 1

_____
_____
_____

Snack 2

_____
_____
_____

Water
Sleep
KCal

What time did you eat? Write B for Breakfast, S1 for Snack 1, S2 for Snack 2, L for Lunch, D for Dinner

5   6   7   8   9   10   11   12   13   14   15   16   17   18   19   20   21   22   23   24+

Physical Activities Minutes / Laps / Sets / ...

- ☐ Fast Walking _____
- ☐ Running _____
- ☐ Aerobics / Zumba _____
- ☐ Yoga / Pilates _____
- ☐ _____
- ☐ _____

Today's Notes

_____
_____

Drugs & Supplements

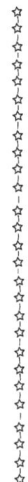

_____
_____
_____

Bad Habits

MOOD

😖 😐 😊

Day 11

Date ___ / ___ / ___

Breakfast

Lunch

Dinner

Snack 1

Snack 2

Water _____

Sleep _____

KCal _____

What time did you eat? Write B for Breakfast, S1 for Snack 1, S2 for Snack 2, L for Lunch, D for Dinner

5	6	7	8	9	10	11	12	13	14	15	16	17	18	19	20	21	22	23	24+

Physical Activities
Minutes / Laps / Sets / ...

- [ ] Fast Walking
- [ ] Running
- [ ] Aerobics / Zumba
- [ ] Yoga / Pilates
- [ ]
- [ ]

Today's Notes

Drugs & Supplements

Bad Habits

MOOD

Day 12

Date ___ / ___ / ___

Breakfast

Lunch

Dinner

Snack 1

Snack 2

- Water
- Sleep
- KCal

What time did you eat? Write B for Breakfast, S1 for Snack 1, S2 for Snack 2, L for Lunch, D for Dinner

5 6 7 8 9 10 11 12 13 14 15 16 17 18 19 20 21 22 23 24+

Physical Activities Minutes / Laps / Sets / ...

- ☐ Fast Walking
- ☐ Running
- ☐ Aerobics / Zumba
- ☐ Yoga / Pilates
- ☐
- ☐

Today's Notes

Drugs & Supplements

Bad Habits

MOOD

Day 13

Date ___ / ___ / ___

Breakfast

_____
_____
_____
_____
_____
_____

Lunch

_____
_____
_____
_____
_____
_____

Dinner

_____
_____
_____
_____
_____
_____

Snack 1

_____
_____
_____

Snack 2

_____
_____
_____

Water _____

Sleep _____

KCal _____

What time did you eat? Write B for Breakfast, S1 for Snack 1, S2 for Snack 2, L for Lunch, D for Dinner

5 6 7 8 9 10 11 12 13 14 15 16 17 18 19 20 21 22 23 24+

Physical Activities Minutes / Laps / Sets / ...

- [ ] Fast Walking
- [ ] Running
- [ ] Aerobics / Zumba
- [ ] Yoga / Pilates
- [ ]
- [ ]

Today's Notes

_____

Drugs & Supplements

_____
_____
_____

Bad Habits

MOOD

Day 14

Date ___/___/___

Breakfast

Lunch

Dinner

Snack 1

Snack 2

Water _____

Sleep _____

KCal _____

What time did you eat? Write B for Breakfast, S1 for Snack 1, S2 for Snack 2, L for Lunch, D for Dinner

5	6	7	8	9	10	11	12	13	14	15	16	17	18	19	20	21	22	23	24+

Physical Activities   Minutes / Laps / Sets / ...

☐ Fast Walking

☐ Running

☐ Aerobics / Zumba

☐ Yoga / Pilates

☐

☐

Today's Notes

Drugs & Supplements

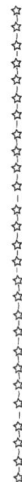

Bad Habits

MOOD

Second Week - Check Point

Review what you wrote this week and answer the questions:

1) How many times have you had a snack between breakfast and lunch?

2) How many times have you had a snack between lunch and dinner?

3) How many times have you eaten fresh fruit as a snack?

If you answered at least 2 to the first question and 2 to the second question, you have reached this week's goal and you can mark a nice "X" on the Week 2 star.
If you answered at least 3 to the third question, then you went beyond the target very good!
If you didn't do it, don't worry, try to understand what prevented you from doing it and we'll try again next week.

Now, if you like, you can write down current weight. Don't worry too much if you feel you're not losing weight fast enough. Remember that rapid descents do not lead to lasting results.
It is better to do things more calmly and get results that last over time!

Weight

_____

♡ ♡ ♡ ♡ ♡ ♡
NOTICE
Keep applying the first and second weeks' advice over the next few weeks until you turn them into habits. Fill in your diary every day, always read the 3 sentences about the right mindset to keep and divide what you eat into 5 meals.

How did the first two weeks go?

_____
_____
_____
_____
_____
_____
_____
_____
_____
_____

Week 3

This week we see "the rule of hands". Using your hands, you can get a quick indication of what the recommended portions are for each type of food.

SALAD AND LEAF VEGETABLES (SPINACH, CHARD, CHICORY, ETC.): THE QUANTITY OF TWO DOUBLE HANDFULS
FRUIT: THE QUANTITY OF TWO CUPPED HANDS (2 TIMES A DAY AT LEAST)

PASTA, RICE, BREAD, POTATOES:
ONE CLENCHED FIST
VEGETABLES: (BROCCOLI, ARTICHOKES, ETC.)
ONE CLENCHED FIST

DRIED FRUITS AND SEEDS:
ONE HANDFUL(MAX 30 GR.) PER DAY

CHOCOLATE: ONE FINGER - **CAKE**: TWO FINGERS

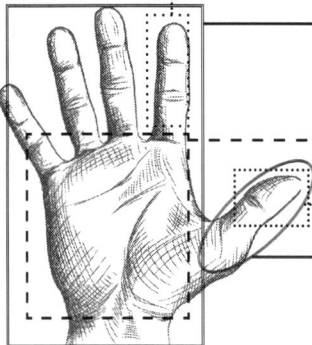

FISH:
A WHOLE HAND, FROM WRIST TO FINGERTIPS

BEEF: ONE PALM (WITHOUT FINGERS)

BUTTER: A THUMB TIP

CHEESE: 2 THUMBS

Small Step of the Week:
IN AT LEAST 3 LUNCHES AND 3 DINNERS:
· USE THE HAND RULE TO MAKE PORTIONS.
GIVE IT A SHOT!

Day (15)

Date ___ / ___ / ___

Breakfast

_____
_____
_____
_____
_____
_____

Lunch

_____
_____
_____
_____
_____
_____

Dinner

_____
_____
_____
_____
_____
_____

Snack 1

_____
_____
_____

Snack 2

_____
_____
_____

Water

Sleep

KCal

What time did you eat? Write B for Breakfast, S1 for Snack 1, S2 for Snack 2, L for Lunch, D for Dinner

5	6	7	8	9	10	11	12	13	14	15	16	17	18	19	20	21	22	23	24+

Physical Activities Minutes / Laps / Sets / ...

☐ Fast Walking
☐ Running
☐ Aerobics / Zumba
☐ Yoga / Pilates
☐
☐

Today's Notes

Drugs & Supplements

Bad Habits

MOOD

😞 😐 😊

It does not matter how slowly you go as long as you do not stop. (Confucius)

Day 16

Date ___ / ___ / ___

Breakfast

Lunch

Dinner

Snack 1

Snack 2

Water

Sleep

KCal

What time did you eat? Write B for Breakfast, S1 for Snack 1, S2 for Snack 2, L for Lunch, D for Dinner

5   6   7   8   9   10   11   12   13   14   15   16   17   18   19   20   21   22   23   24+

Physical Activities   Minutes / Laps / Sets / ...

- [ ] Fast Walking
- [ ] Running
- [ ] Aerobics / Zumba
- [ ] Yoga / Pilates
- [ ]
- [ ]

Today's Notes

Drugs & Supplements

Bad Habits

MOOD

Don't worry about finding stop signs,
start moving now and you will find the way to get anywhere you want. (Anon.)

Day (17)

Date _____ / _____ / _____

Breakfast

Lunch

Dinner

....
....
....
....
....
....

Snack 1

Snack 2

....
....
....

Water _____

Sleep _____

KCal _____

What time did you eat? Write B for Breakfast, S1 for Snack 1, S2 for Snack 2, L for Lunch, D for Dinner

| 5 | 6 | 7 | 8 | 9 | 10 | 11 | 12 | 13 | 14 | 15 | 16 | 17 | 18 | 19 | 20 | 21 | 22 | 23 | 24+ |

Physical Activities Minutes / Laps / Sets / ...

- ☐ Fast Walking
- ☐ Running
- ☐ Aerobics / Zumba
- ☐ Yoga / Pilates
- ☐
- ☐

Today's Notes

Drugs & Supplements

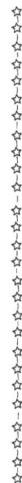

Bad Habits

MOOD

If you can dream it, you can do it. The secret is to start moving. (Walt Disney)

Day 18

Date ___ / ___ / ___

Breakfast

Lunch

Dinner

Snack 1

Snack 2

Water _____

Sleep _____

KCal _____

What time did you eat? Write B for Breakfast, S1 for Snack 1, S2 for Snack 2, L for Lunch, D for Dinner

| 5 | 6 | 7 | 8 | 9 | 10 | 11 | 12 | 13 | 14 | 15 | 16 | 17 | 18 | 19 | 20 | 21 | 22 | 23 | 24+ |

♥ Physical Activities   Minutes / Laps / Sets / ...

- ☐ Fast Walking
- ☐ Running
- ☐ Aerobics / Zumba
- ☐ Yoga / Pilates
- ☐
- ☐

🍃 Today's Notes

💊 Drugs & Supplements

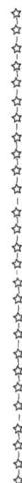

🚭 Bad Habits

MOOD

Day 19

Date ___ / ___ / ___

Breakfast

_____
_____
_____
_____
_____
_____
_____
_____

Lunch

_____
_____
_____
_____
_____
_____
_____
_____

Dinner

_____
_____
_____
_____
_____
_____
_____
_____

Snack 1

_____
_____
_____

Snack 2

_____
_____
_____

Water _____

Sleep _____

KCal _____

What time did you eat? Write B for Breakfast, S1 for Snack 1, S2 for Snack 2, L for Lunch, D for Dinner

5	6	7	8	9	10	11	12	13	14	15	16	17	18	19	20	21	22	23	24+

Physical Activities Minutes / Laps / Sets / ...

- ☐ Fast Walking ....
- ☐ Running ....
- ☐ Aerobics / Zumba ....
- ☐ Yoga / Pilates ....
- ☐ ....
- ☐ ....

Today's Notes

_____

Drugs & Supplements

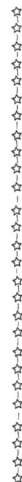

_____
_____
_____

Bad Habits

MOOD

Challenges are what make life interesting; overcoming them is what makes life meaningful.
(JJ Marine)

Day 20   Date ___ / ___ / ___

Breakfast
_____
_____
_____
_____
_____
_____
_____
_____

Snack 1
_____
_____
_____
_____

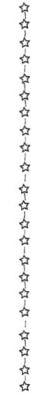

Lunch
_____
_____
_____
_____
_____
_____
_____
_____

Snack 2
_____
_____
_____
_____

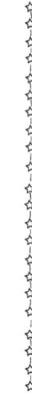

Dinner
_____
_____
_____
_____
_____
_____
_____
_____

🥛 Water _____

🕐 Sleep _____

KCal _____

What time did you eat? Write B for Breakfast, S1 for Snack 1, S2 for Snack 2, L for Lunch, D for Dinner

5   6   7   8   9   10   11   12   13   14   15   16   17   18   19   20   21   22   23   24+

❤ Physical Activities   Minutes / Laps / Sets / ...

☐ Fast Walking   _____
☐ Running   _____
☐ Aerobics / Zumba   _____
☐ Yoga / Pilates   _____
☐ _____   _____
☐ _____   _____

🌿 Today's Notes
_____
_____
_____

Drugs & Supplements
_____
_____
_____

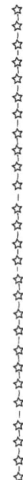

Bad Habits

🚭   🍸

🍰   ☕

MOOD
☹   😐   😊

There is only one corner of the universe you can be certain of improving, and that's your own self.
(A. Huxley)

Day 21

Date ___ / ___ / ___

Breakfast

Lunch

Dinner

Snack 1

Snack 2

- Water _____
- Sleep _____
- KCal _____

What time did you eat? Write B for Breakfast, S1 for Snack 1, S2 for Snack 2, L for Lunch, D for Dinner

| 5 | 6 | 7 | 8 | 9 | 10 | 11 | 12 | 13 | 14 | 15 | 16 | 17 | 18 | 19 | 20 | 21 | 22 | 23 | 24+ |

Physical Activities *Minutes / Laps / Sets / ...*

- ☐ Fast Walking _____
- ☐ Running _____
- ☐ Aerobics / Zumba _____
- ☐ Yoga / Pilates _____
- ☐ _____
- ☐ _____

Drugs & Supplements

Bad Habits

Today's Notes

MOOD

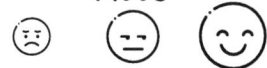

Start where you are. Use what you have. Do what you can. (Arthur Ashe)

Third Week - Check Point

Review what you wrote this week and answer the questions:

1) In how many lunches or dinners have you used the hand rule to make portions?

2) Were you able to eat only the amount required by the "rule of hands"?

If you answered at least 3 to the first question, you have reached this week's goal and you can mark a nice "X" on the Week 3 star.

If you answered "YES" to the second question, then you went beyond the target very good!

If you didn't do it, don't worry, try to understand what prevented you from doing it and we'll try again next week.

Now, if you like, you can write down current weight. If you have not reached the weight you expected do not be discouraged, you have everything you need in front of you to be able to change things immediately and within you. You have the strength to do it, let it out and the results will come.

Weight

_____

♡ ♡ ♡ ♡ ♡ ♡

NOTICE

As you try to apply the advice of the new week, continue to follow those of the previous weeks as well, fill in your diary every day and always read the 3 sentences about the right mindset to maintain

How did the first three weeks go?

_____

_____

_____

_____

_____

_____

_____

_____

_____

_____

_____

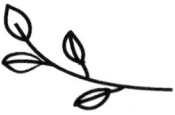

Week 4

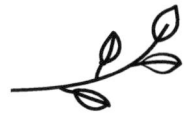

Last week we saw how important portions are, but to provide our body with all the elements it needs we must follow a balanced diet in all its components. To do this we must eat every day, both for lunch and dinner, foods that offer us carbohydrates, proteins, fats, fibers and vitamins in the right proportions.
Don't worry if it seems like a difficult thing to do, the "HEALTHY DISH RULE" comes to your aid.

This rule says that our dish must be composed like this:

*   **25 %** Pasta, Grain Cereals, Bread o Potatoes
*   **25 %** Meat, Fish, Eggs o Cheeses
*   **35 %** Cooked or Raw Vegetables
*   **15 %** Fresh Fruit
    *

It is not necessary that these components are eaten separately, you can create unique dishes (for example: Rice, Zucchini and Shrimp or Spaghetti, Tomatoes and Mozzarella) or create a dish with a second course (for example: meat, fish or eggs) accompanied by a vegetable side dish and a slice of bread.

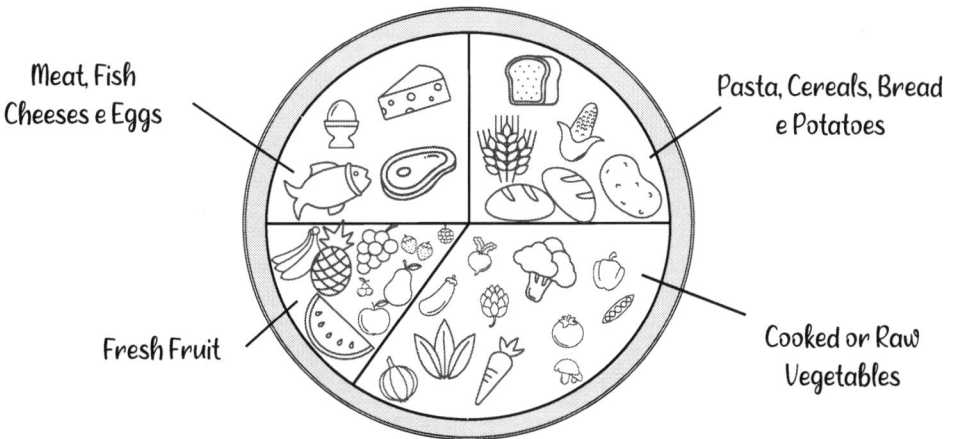

Meat, Fish Cheeses e Eggs

Pasta, Cereals, Bread e Potatoes

Fresh Fruit

Cooked or Raw Vegetables

Small Step of the Week:
MAKE 3 LAUNCHES AND 3 DINNERS FOLLOWING THE HEALTHY "DISH RULE"
GIVE IT A TRY!

Day 22

Date _____ / _____ / _____

Breakfast

Lunch

Dinner

Snack 1

Snack 2

Water

Sleep

KCal

What time did you eat? Write B for Breakfast, S1 for Snack 1, S2 for Snack 2, L for Lunch, D for Dinner

| 5 | 6 | 7 | 8 | 9 | 10 | 11 | 12 | 13 | 14 | 15 | 16 | 17 | 18 | 19 | 20 | 21 | 22 | 23 | 24+ |

Physical Activities Minutes / Laps / Sets / ...

- [ ] Fast Walking
- [ ] Running
- [ ] Aerobics / Zumba
- [ ] Yoga / Pilates
- [ ]
- [ ]

Today's Notes

Drugs & Supplements

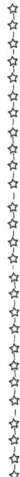

Bad Habits

MOOD

Step by step and the thing is done. (Charles Atlas)

Day 23

Date ___ / ___ / ___

Breakfast

_____
_____
_____
_____
_____
_____
_____

Lunch

_____
_____
_____
_____
_____
_____
_____

Dinner

_____
_____
_____
_____
_____
_____
_____

Snack 1

_____
_____
_____
_____

Snack 2

_____
_____
_____
_____

Water _____

Sleep _____

KCal _____

What time did you eat? Write B for Breakfast, S1 for Snack 1, S2 for Snack 2, L for Lunch, D for Dinner

5   6   7   8   9   10   11   12   13   14   15   16   17   18   19   20   21   22   23   24+

Physical Activities Minutes / Laps / Sets / ...

☐ Fast Walking _____
☐ Running _____
☐ Aerobics / Zumba _____
☐ Yoga / Pilates _____
☐ _____
☐ _____

Today's Notes

_____

Drugs & Supplements

_____
_____
_____

Bad Habits

MOOD

Don't wait until everything is perfect before taking action, just do it.

Day 24

Date _____ / _____ / _____

Breakfast
_____
_____
_____
_____
_____
_____
_____

Lunch
_____
_____
_____
_____
_____
_____
_____

Dinner
_____
_____
_____
_____
_____
_____
_____

Snack 1
_____
_____
_____

Snack 2
_____
_____
_____

Water _____
Sleep _____
KCal _____

What time did you eat? Write B for Breakfast, S1 for Snack 1, S2 for Snack 2, L for Lunch, D for Dinner

5	6	7	8	9	10	11	12	13	14	15	16	17	18	19	20	21	22	23	24+

Physical Activities Minutes / Laps / Sets / ...

- ☐ Fast Walking _____
- ☐ Running _____
- ☐ Aerobics / Zumba _____
- ☐ Yoga / Pilates _____
- ☐ _____
- ☐ _____

Today's Notes
_____
_____

Drugs & Supplements
_____
_____

Bad Habits

MOOD
☹ 😐 🙂

Don't give up, a stone at the time builds a castle.

Day 25

Date ___ / ___ / ___

Breakfast

Lunch

Dinner

Snack 1

Snack 2

Water ___

Sleep ___

KCal ___

What time did you eat? Write B for Breakfast, S1 for Snack 1, S2 for Snack 2, L for Lunch, D for Dinner

5	6	7	8	9	10	11	12	13	14	15	16	17	18	19	20	21	22	23	24+

Physical Activities Minutes / Laps / Sets / ...

- [ ] Fast Walking
- [ ] Running
- [ ] Aerobics / Zumba
- [ ] Yoga / Pilates
- [ ]
- [ ]

Drugs & Supplements

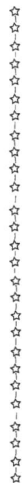

Bad Habits

Today's Notes

MOOD

Day 26

Date ___/___/___

Breakfast

_____
_____
_____
_____
_____
_____
_____
_____

Lunch

_____
_____
_____
_____
_____
_____
_____
_____

Dinner

_____
_____
_____
_____
_____
_____
_____
_____

Snack 1

_____
_____
_____
_____

Snack 2

_____
_____
_____
_____

Water _____

Sleep _____

KCal _____

What time did you eat? Write B for Breakfast, S1 for Snack 1, S2 for Snack 2, L for Lunch, D for Dinner

5 6 7 8 9 10 11 12 13 14 15 16 17 18 19 20 21 22 23 24+

Physical Activities Minutes / Laps / Sets / ...

- ☐ Fast Walking _____
- ☐ Running _____
- ☐ Aerobics / Zumba _____
- ☐ Yoga / Pilates _____
- ☐ _____
- ☐ _____

Today's Notes

_____
_____

Drugs & Supplements

_____
_____
_____

Bad Habits

MOOD

☹ 😐 🙂

Day 27

Date ___ / ___ / ___

Breakfast

Lunch

Dinner

Snack 1

Snack 2

Water _____

Sleep _____

KCal _____

What time did you eat? Write B for Breakfast, S1 for Snack 1, S2 for Snack 2, L for Lunch, D for Dinner

5   6   7   8   9   10   11   12   13   14   15   16   17   18   19   20   21   22   23   24+

Physical Activities   Minutes / Laps / Sets / ...

- [ ] Fast Walking
- [ ] Running
- [ ] Aerobics / Zumba
- [ ] Yoga / Pilates
- [ ]
- [ ]

Today's Notes

Drugs & Supplements

Bad Habits

MOOD

Day 28

Date _____ / _____ / _____

Breakfast

Lunch

Dinner

Snack 1

Snack 2

Water

Sleep

KCal

Write B for Breakfast, S1 for Snack 1, S2 for Snack 2, L for Lunch, D for Dinner

5   6   7   8   9   10   11   12   13   14   15   16   17   18   19   20   21   22   23   24+

Physical Activities   Minutes / Laps / Sets / ...

- [ ] Fast Walking
- [ ] Running
- [ ] Aerobics / Zumba
- [ ] Yoga / Pilates
- [ ]
- [ ]

Drugs & Supplements

Bad Habits

Today's Notes

MOOD

Fourth Week Check Point

Review what you wrote this week and answer the questions:

1) How many times have you followed the healthy meal rule for lunch?

2) How many times have you followed the healthy meal rule for dinner?

If you answered at least 3 to the first question and 3 to the second question, you have reached this week's goal and you can mark a nice "X" on the Week 4 Star.
If you didn't do it, don't worry, try to understand what prevented you from doing it and we'll try again next week.

♡ ♡ ♡ ♡ ♡ ♡ Do we take measurements? ♡ ♡ ♡ ♡ ♡ ♡

Date _____

Neck _____

Bust _____

Arms _____

Waist _____

Abdomen _____

Hips _____

Thighs _____

Upper Knee _____

Calf _____

Weight _____

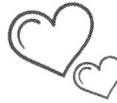

How did the first four weeks go?

_____

_____

_____

_____

_____

_____

_____

_____

Remember that to change your habits it takes a lot of patience and a lot of perseverance. These will be your winning weapons on this path. If you can't stick to your diet for a few days, don't beat yourself up, it's normal. You must never think that a few wasted days make what you have already done useless.

You have to be proud of yourself for every little step you take.

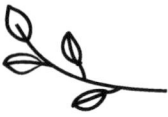

Week 5

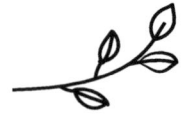

Before we get to your little step of the week we will dispel the false belief that carbohydrates should be avoided because they "make you gain weight".
Carbohydrates, in fact, are the main source of the energy our body needs and we must take eat them at least twice a day, every day, in the right quantities.

The foods that contain the greatest amount of carbohydrates are those that derive from cereals (wheat, rice, corn, barley, spelled, ...) and pseudo-cereals (buckwheat, quinoa, amaranth).
Whole Grains and Pseudo Grains have greater satiating power than refined grains and are an excellent source of fiber.

Try to gradually replace refined grains with whole grains because:

• They are richer in fiber, vitamins and minerals
• They improve the functioning of the intestine
• Lower cholesterol levels
• They help prevent the onset of diabetes and cardiovascular diseases
• They have an antitumor function
• Reduce the sense of hunger
• Help to keep weight under control
• They are tastier

Small Step of the week:

EAT, IN AT LEAST 3 DIFFERENT DAYS, WHOLEMEAL PRODUCTS INSTEAD OF THE "CLASSIC" ONES.

GIVE IT A SHOT!

Day 29

Date _____ / _____ / _____

Breakfast

Lunch

Dinner

Snack 1

Snack 2

💧 Water _____

🕐 Sleep _____

🍽 KCal _____

What time did you eat? Write B for Breakfast, S1 for Snack 1, S2 for Snack 2, L for Lunch, D for Dinner

5	6	7	8	9	10	11	12	13	14	15	16	17	18	19	20	21	22	23	24+

Physical Activities Minutes / Laps / Sets / ...

- ☐ Fast Walking
- ☐ Running
- ☐ Aerobics / Zumba
- ☐ Yoga / Pilates
- ☐
- ☐

Today's Notes

Drugs & Supplements

Bad Habits

MOOD

☹ 😐 🙂

If last week wasn't exactly how you wanted it to be, this one will certainly be better.

Day 30

Date _____ / _____ / _____

Breakfast

_____
_____
_____
_____
_____
_____
_____

Lunch

_____
_____
_____
_____
_____
_____
_____

Dinner

_____
_____
_____
_____
_____
_____
_____

Snack 1

_____
_____
_____

Snack 2

_____
_____
_____

- Water
- Sleep
- KCal

What time did you eat? Write B for Breakfast, S1 for Snack 1, S2 for Snack 2, L for Lunch, D for Dinner

5   6   7   8   9   10   11   12   13   14   15   16   17   18   19   20   21   22   23   24+

Physical Activities Minutes / Laps / Sets / ...

- ☐ Fast Walking   _____
- ☐ Running   _____
- ☐ Aerobics / Zumba _____
- ☐ Yoga / Pilates _____
- ☐   _____
- ☐   _____

Drugs & Supplements

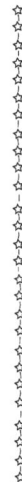

_____
_____
_____

Bad Habits

MOOD

(☹)   (😐)   (☺)

Today's Notes

_____
_____
_____

In optimism there is magic. In pessimism there is nothing. (Abraham-Hicks)

Day 31

Date ___ / ___ / ___

Breakfast

Lunch

Dinner

Snack 1

Snack 2

Water _____

Sleep _____

KCal _____

What time did you eat? Write B for Breakfast, S1 for Snack 1, S2 for Snack 2, L for Lunch, D for Dinner

| 5 | 6 | 7 | 8 | 9 | 10 | 11 | 12 | 13 | 14 | 15 | 16 | 17 | 18 | 19 | 20 | 21 | 22 | 23 | 24+ |

Physical Activities Minutes / Laps / Sets / …

- [ ] Fast Walking
- [ ] Running
- [ ] Aerobics / Zumba
- [ ] Yoga / Pilates
- [ ]
- [ ]

Today's Notes

Drugs & Supplements

Bad Habits

MOOD

Day 32

Date ___ / ___ / ___

Breakfast

_____
_____
_____
_____
_____
_____
_____

Lunch

_____
_____
_____
_____
_____
_____
_____

Dinner

_____
_____
_____
_____
_____
_____
_____

Snack 1

_____
_____
_____

Snack 2

_____
_____
_____

Water _____

Sleep _____

KCal _____

What time did you eat? Write B for Breakfast, S1 for Snack 1, S2 for Snack 2, L for Lunch, D for Dinner

5	6	7	8	9	10	11	12	13	14	15	16	17	18	19	20	21	22	23	24+

Physical Activities Minutes / Laps / Sets / ...

- [ ] Fast Walking _____
- [ ] Running _____
- [ ] Aerobics / Zumba _____
- [ ] Yoga / Pilates _____
- [ ] _____
- [ ] _____

Today's Notes

_____
_____
_____

Drugs & Supplements

_____
_____
_____

Bad Habits

MOOD

Setting goals is the first step in turning the invisible into the visible. (A. Robbins)

Day 33

Date ___ / ___ / ___

Breakfast

Lunch

Dinner

Snack 1

Snack 2

Water

Sleep

KCal

What time did you eat? Write B for Breakfast, S1 for Snack 1, S2 for Snack 2, L for Lunch, D for Dinner

5	6	7	8	9	10	11	12	13	14	15	16	17	18	19	20	21	22	23	24+

Physical Activities   Minutes / Laps / Sets / ...

- ☐ Fast Walking
- ☐ Running
- ☐ Aerobics / Zumba
- ☐ Yoga / Pilates
- ☐
- ☐

Today's Notes

Drugs & Supplements

Bad Habits

MOOD

Day 34

Date .... / /

Breakfast

Lunch

Dinner

Snack 1

Snack 2

Water

Sleep

KCal

What time did you eat? Write B for Breakfast, S1 for Snack 1, S2 for Snack 2, L for Lunch, D for Dinner

| 5 | 6 | 7 | 8 | 9 | 10 | 11 | 12 | 13 | 14 | 15 | 16 | 17 | 18 | 19 | 20 | 21 | 22 | 23 | 24+ |

Physical Activities Minutes / Laps / Sets / ...

- [ ] Fast Walking
- [ ] Running
- [ ] Aerobics / Zumba
- [ ] Yoga / Pilates
- [ ]
- [ ]

Today's Notes

Drugs & Supplements

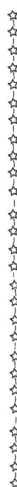

Bad Habits

MOOD

Day (35)

Date ____ / ____ / ____

Breakfast	Lunch	Dinner

Snack 1

Snack 2

Water ____

Sleep ____

KCal ____

What time did you eat? Write B for Breakfast, S1 for Snack 1, S2 for Snack 2, L for Lunch, D for Dinner

5 6 7 8 9 10 11 12 13 14 15 16 17 18 19 20 21 22 23 24+

Physical Activities Minutes / Laps / Sets / ...

- ☐ Fast Walking
- ☐ Running
- ☐ Aerobics / Zumba
- ☐ Yoga / Pilates
- ☐
- ☐

Today's Notes

Drugs & Supplements

Bad Habits

MOOD

Fifth Week Check Point:

Review what you wrote this week and answer the questions:

1) How many times have you eaten whole grains for lunch?

2) How many times have you eaten whole grains for dinner?

If the sum of your answers is at least 6 you have reached this week's goal and you can mark a nice "X" on the Week 5 Star.

Whole grains are excellent ingredients for preparing unique healthy and balanced dishes. You can try to make a mix of spelled, barley and buckwheat, add cherry tomatoes and zucchini, a few cubes of Feta and two chopped walnuts. You will have made a very colorful and above all very nutritious dish.

Now, if you like, you can write down your current weight. Whatever the result is, don't be too influenced by it.
If it's positive, celebrate!

If it isn't, don't get discouraged because it just means you need a little more time. Only those who give up do not reach the finish line, and you don't want to give up, do you?

Weight _____

How did the first 5 weeks go?

♥ ♥ ♥ ♥ ♥ ♥
NOTICE
Keep applying the advice from previous weeks as you strive to take the new little step. Fill in your Diary every day and re-read the sentences on the right mindset to maintain. A positive attitude will be your winning weapon.

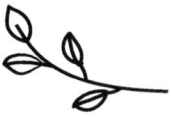

Week 6

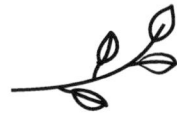

This week we focus on one small step that can give you so many benefits that we can consider it as almost the most important one of all, and it is not as difficult to do as you might think: Exercise.

You often give up on physical activity for lack of time, but you can use some tricks to incorporate it into your day. To get the benefits that exercise can give you, 30 minutes a day are enough, and you can divide this time into Intervals.

For example: if you go to work by car you can park 15 minutes away from your office and reach it with a brisk walk, or if you are traveling by public transportation you can get off a few stops before your destination. This way you did your daily 30 minutes almost without realizing it.

Physical activity, even if it's light, has the ability to improve your general well-being because, in addition to being good for the body, it is good for the mind. Physical activity stimulates the body to produce endorphins, the famous "hormone of happiness".
Try wearing a pair of headphones, play your favorite songs and dance for 10 minutes, the effect it will have on your mood will be great.

Small Step of the Week:
DO AT LEAST 30 MINUTES OF PHYSICAL ACTIVITY A DAY, ON 3 DIFFERENT DAYS
GIVE IT A TRY!

Day 36

Date ____ / ____ / ____

Breakfast

Lunch

Dinner

Snack 1

Snack 2

Water ____
Sleep ____
KCal ____

What time did you eat? Write B for Breakfast, S1 for Snack 1, S2 for Snack 2, L for Lunch, D for Dinner

5   6   7   8   9   10   11   12   13   14   15   16   17   18   19   20   21   22   23   24+

Physical Activities Minutes / Laps / Sets / ...

- [ ] Fast Walking ____
- [ ] Running ____
- [ ] Aerobics / Zumba ____
- [ ] Yoga / Pilates ____
- [ ] ____
- [ ] ____

Drugs & Supplements

Today's Notes

Bad Habits

MOOD

Day 37

Date ___ / ___ / ___

Breakfast

Lunch

Dinner

Snack 1

Snack 2

Water

Sleep

KCal

What time did you eat? Write B for Breakfast, S1 for Snack 1, S2 for Snack 2, L for Lunch, D for Dinner

5   6   7   8   9   10   11   12   13   14   15   16   17   18   19   20   21   22   23   24+

Physical Activities   Minutes / Laps / Sets / ...

☐ Fast Walking

☐ Running

☐ Aerobics / Zumba

☐ Yoga / Pilates

☐

☐

Today's Notes

Drugs & Supplements

Bad Habits

MOOD

It's only when the "one day's" become "now's" that dreams become reality. (A. Robbins)

Day 38

Date ___ /___ /___

Breakfast

_____
_____
_____
_____
_____
_____
_____
_____

Lunch

_____
_____
_____
_____
_____
_____
_____
_____

Dinner

_____
_____
_____
_____
_____
_____
_____
_____

Snack 1

_____
_____
_____

Snack 2

_____
_____
_____

Water _____

Sleep _____

KCal _____

What time did you eat? Write B for Breakfast, S1 for Snack 1, S2 for Snack 2, L for Lunch, D for Dinner

5   6   7   8   9   10   11   12   13   14   15   16   17   18   19   20   21   22   23   24+

Physical Activities Minutes / Laps / Sets / ...

- [ ] Fast Walking _____
- [ ] Running _____
- [ ] Aerobics / Zumba _____
- [ ] Yoga / Pilates _____
- [ ] _____
- [ ] _____

Drugs & Supplements

_____
_____
_____
_____

Bad Habits

Today's Notes

_____
_____

MOOD

The world lies in the hands of those that have the courage to dream and who take the risk of living out their dreams. (Paulo Coelho)

Day 39

Date ___ / ___ / ___

Breakfast

Lunch

Dinner

Snack 1

Snack 2

Water ___

Sleep ___

KCal ___

What time did you eat? Write B for Breakfast, S1 for Snack 1, S2 for Snack 2, L for Lunch, D for Dinner

5 6 7 8 9 10 11 12 13 14 15 16 17 18 19 20 21 22 23 24+

Physical Activities Minutes / Laps / Sets / ...

- ☐ Fast Walking
- ☐ Running
- ☐ Aerobics / Zumba
- ☐ Yoga / Pilates
- ☐
- ☐

Today's Notes

Drugs & Supplements

Bad Habits

MOOD

Day 40

Date ___ / ___ / ___

Breakfast

Lunch

Dinner

Snack 1

Snack 2

🥤 Water

😴 Sleep

🍽 KCal

What time did you eat? Write B for Breakfast, S1 for Snack 1, S2 for Snack 2, L for Lunch, D for Dinner

5   6   7   8   9   10   11   12   13   14   15   16   17   18   19   20   21   22   23   24+

❤ Physical Activities   Minutes / Laps / Sets / ...

Drugs & Supplements

☐ Fast Walking

☐ Running

☐ Aerobics / Zumba

☐ Yoga / Pilates

☐

☐

🚫 Bad Habits

🍃 Today's Notes

MOOD

☹ 😐 🙂

Today take a decision you have always put off, and tomorrow take.... (continue in the next page)

Day (41)   Date ___ / ___ / ___

Breakfast

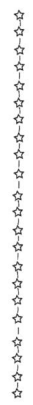

Lunch

Dinner

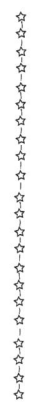

Snack 1

Snack 2

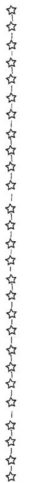

Water
Sleep
KCal

What time did you eat? Write B for Breakfast, S1 for Snack 1, S2 for Snack 2, L for Lunch, D for Dinner

5 6 7 8 9 10 11 12 13 14 15 16 17 18 19 20 21 22 23 24+

Physical Activities   Minutes / Laps / Sets / ...

- ☐ Fast Walking
- ☐ Running
- ☐ Aerobics / Zumba
- ☐ Yoga / Pilates
- ☐
- ☐

Today's Notes

Drugs & Supplements

Bad Habits

MOOD

😣 😑 😊

Day 42

Date ___ / ___ / ___

Breakfast

Lunch

Dinner

Snack 1

Snack 2

Water _____

Sleep _____

KCal _____

What time did you eat? Write B for Breakfast, S1 for Snack 1, S2 for Snack 2, L for Lunch, D for Dinner

5 6 7 8 9 10 11 12 13 14 15 16 17 18 19 20 21 22 23 24+

Physical Activities Minutes / Laps / Sets / ...

- ☐ Fast Walking
- ☐ Running
- ☐ Aerobics / Zumba
- ☐ Yoga / Pilates
- ☐
- ☐

Today's Notes

Drugs & Supplements

Bad Habits

MOOD

Sixth Week Check Point:

Review what you wrote this week and answer the questions:

1) How many times have you done 30 minutes of physical activity?

2) How many times have you tried to lengthen the routes you had to walk?

If you answered at least 3 to the first question, you have reached this week's goal and you can mark a nice "X" on the star of Week 6. If you answered at least 2 to the second, then you have also gone beyond the goal, very good! If you didn't do it, don't worry, try to understand what prevented you from doing it and we'll try again next week.

If you can already do at least half an hour of physical activity 3 times a week you can try to increase your commitment. For a healthy adult, about two and a half to three hours of physical activity a week are ideal for keeping in perfect shape, keeping weight under control and drastically reducing the risk of cardiovascular disease. It is not essential to join the gym, just a little space at home, a video workout on YouTube and we have everything we need to get started.

Don't wait for the perfect time to start, The right time is NOW.

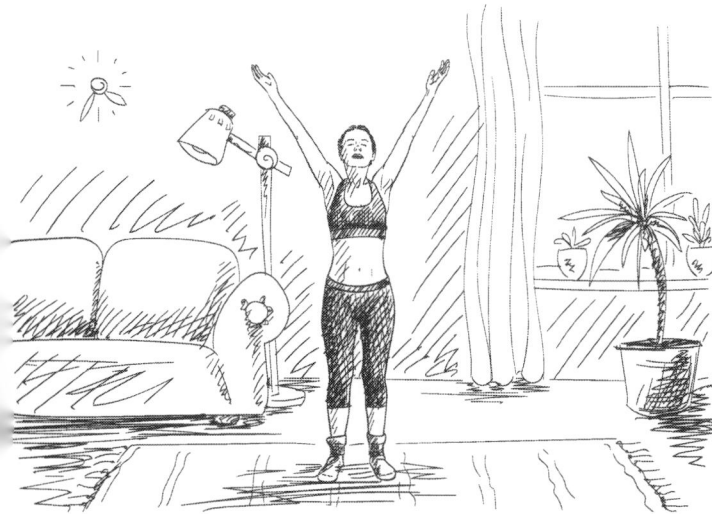

Now, if you like, you can write down your current weight. Remember that it is more important to have taken a step towards your goal than the number you read on the scale.

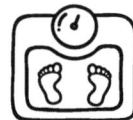

Weight:
_____

Notes:

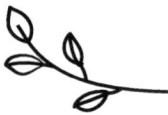

Week 7

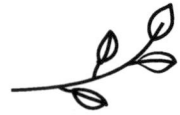

If you are among those who run away in a flash in the morning and do not eat anything this week, I have some advice for you.

Breakfast is the most important meal of the day because it allows us to set our diet correctly from the morning: if we wake up and we have a good breakfast, we will feel satisfied for several hours, and starting to feel hunger again at the right time to have a snack. If we skip breakfast, we risk finding ourselves too close to lunch eating very caloric foods, and these will end up ruining our lunch too, and so on until dinner.

Breakfast, as well as lunch and dinner, should be well balanced, meaning it should provide you with carbohydrates, proteins and fats.

It is possible to obtain a balanced breakfast whether you prefer it "sweet" or whether you prefer it "salty". For example:

- Sweet breakfast: Milk or Yogurt + Whole Grains + dried fruit
- Savory breakfast: wholemeal bread + 2 eggs + a juice

Avoid having breakfast with croissants, cakes or pastries because they are too caloric and do not give a sense of satiety.

Also avoid sandwiches because they are too high in fat.

Small Step of the week:

IN AT LEAST 3 DIFFERENT DAYS:
EAT A HEALTHY AND BALANCED BREAKFAST
DO NOT EAT CROISSANTS, CAKES OR PIZZAS FOR BREAKFAST
GIVE IT A SHOT!

Consuming a healthy and balanced breakfast calmly can have an incredible effect on the rest of the day, also improving productivity at work or while you study.

Day 43

Date ___/___/___

Breakfast

Lunch

Dinner

Snack 1

Snack 2

Water

Sleep

KCal

What time did you eat? Write B for Breakfast, S1 for Snack 1, S2 for Snack 2, L for Lunch, D for Dinner

5   6   7   8   9   10   11   12   13   14   15   16   17   18   19   20   21   22   23   24+

Physical Activities   Minutes / Laps / Sets / ...

☐ Fast Walking

☐ Running

☐ Aerobics / Zumba

☐ Yoga / Pilates

☐

☐

Drugs & Supplements

Bad Habits

Today's Notes

MOOD

The distance between your dreams and reality is called action.

Day 44

Date ___/___/___

Breakfast

_____
_____
_____
_____
_____
_____

Lunch

_____
_____
_____
_____
_____
_____

Dinner

_____
_____
_____
_____
_____
_____

Snack 1

_____
_____
_____

Snack 2

_____
_____
_____

Water _____

Sleep _____

KCal _____

What time did you eat? Write B for Breakfast, S1 for Snack 1, S2 for Snack 2, L for Lunch, D for Dinner

5	6	7	8	9	10	11	12	13	14	15	16	17	18	19	20	21	22	23	24+

Physical Activities Minutes / Laps / Sets / ...

☐ Fast Walking ....
☐ Running ....
☐ Aerobics / Zumba ....
☐ Yoga / Pilates ....
☐ _____ ....
☐ _____ ....

Today's Notes

_____
_____

Drugs & Supplements

_____
_____
_____
_____

Bad Habits

MOOD

Never let the things you can't do stop you from doing what you can. (R. Reagan)

Day 45

Date ___ / ___ / ___

Breakfast

Lunch

Dinner

Snack 1

Snack 2

Water ___

Sleep ___

KCal ___

What time did you eat? Write B for Breakfast, S1 for Snack 1, S2 for Snack 2, L for Lunch, D for Dinner

5   6   7   8   9   10   11   12   13   14   15   16   17   18   19   20   21   22   23   24+

Physical Activities Minutes / Laps / Sets / ...

- [ ] Fast Walking
- [ ] Running
- [ ] Aerobics / Zumba
- [ ] Yoga / Pilates
- [ ]
- [ ]

Today's Notes

Drugs & Supplements

Bad Habits

MOOD

I can accept failure, everyone fails at something. But I can't accept not trying. (M. Jordan)

Day (46)

Date ___ / ___ / ___

Breakfast

_____
_____
_____
_____
_____
_____

Lunch

_____
_____
_____
_____
_____
_____

Dinner

_____
_____
_____
_____
_____
_____

Snack 1

_____
_____
_____

Snack 2

_____
_____
_____

Water _____

Sleep _____

KCal _____

What time did you eat? Write B for Breakfast, S1 for Snack 1, S2 for Snack 2, L for Lunch, D for Dinner

5 6 7 8 9 10 11 12 13 14 15 16 17 18 19 20 21 22 23 24+

Physical Activities Minutes / Laps / Sets / ...

- ☐ Fast Walking _____
- ☐ Running _____
- ☐ Aerobics / Zumba _____
- ☐ Yoga / Pilates _____
- ☐ _____
- ☐ _____

Today's Notes

_____
_____
_____

Drugs & Supplements

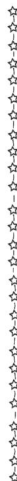

_____
_____
_____
_____

Bad Habits

MOOD

Day (47) Date ___ / ___ / ___

Breakfast

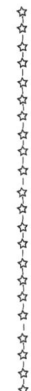

Lunch

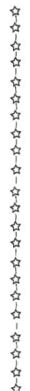

Dinner

Snack 1

Snack 2

Water	___
Sleep	___
KCal	___

What time did you eat? Write B for Breakfast, S1 for Snack 1, S2 for Snack 2, L for Lunch, D for Dinner

5   6   7   8   9   10   11   12   13   14   15   16   17   18   19   20   21   22   23   24+

❤ Physical Activities Minutes / Laps / Sets / ...

- ☐ Fast Walking
- ☐ Running
- ☐ Aerobics / Zumba
- ☐ Yoga / Pilates
- ☐
- ☐

🍃 Today's Notes

Drugs & Supplements

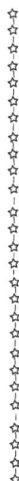

Bad Habits

MOOD

😞 😐 🙂

Some dream to reach their goals. Others work for them.

Day 48

Date ___ / ___ / ___

Breakfast
....
....
....
....
....
....
....

Lunch
....
....
....
....
....
....
....

Dinner
....
....
....
....
....
....
....

Snack 1
....
....
....
....

Snack 2
....
....
....
....

Water _____
Sleep _____
KCal _____

What time did you eat? Write B for Breakfast, S1 for Snack 1, S2 for Snack 2, L for Lunch, D for Dinner

| 5 | 6 | 7 | 8 | 9 | 10 | 11 | 12 | 13 | 14 | 15 | 16 | 17 | 18 | 19 | 20 | 21 | 22 | 23 | 24+ |

Physical Activities Minutes / Laps / Sets / ...

☐ Fast Walking ....
☐ Running ....
☐ Aerobics / Zumba ....
☐ Yoga / Pilates ....
☐ ....
☐ ....

Today's Notes
....
....
....
....

Drugs & Supplements
....
....
....
....

Bad Habits

MOOD
☹ 😐 🙂

Day 49

Date ___ / ___ / ___

Breakfast

Lunch

Dinner

Snack 1

Snack 2

Water _____

Sleep _____

KCal _____

What time did you eat? Write B for Breakfast, S1 for Snack 1, S2 for Snack 2, L for Lunch, D for Dinner

5   6   7   8   9   10   11   12   13   14   15   16   17   18   19   20   21   22   23   24+

Physical Activities Minutes / Laps / Sets / ...

☐ Fast Walking

☐ Running

☐ Aerobics / Zumba

☐ Yoga / Pilates

☐

☐

Today's Notes

Drugs & Supplements

Bad Habits

MOOD

Don't wait for the right moment to act, the only right moment is now.

Seventh Week Check Point:

Review what you wrote this week and answer the questions:

1) How many times have you had a healthy and balanced breakfast?

2) How many times have you had breakfast with pastries or sweets?

3) How many times have you eaten breakfast without rushing?

If you answered at least 3 to the first and third questions you have reached this week's goal and can mark a nice "X" on the Week 7 star. If you answered less than 2 to the third question, then you went beyond the target, very good!
If you didn't do it, don't worry, try to understand what prevented you from doing it and we'll try again next week.

Several studies have shown that having a healthy and balanced breakfast can improve mood and allows us to start the day in a great way.
You can use the holidays to try something new for breakfast for example you could try making pancakes with rice flour, accompanied by blueberries.
Finally, jam is also good for breakfast, but choose the one with no added sugar.

♡ ♡ ♡ ♡ ♡ ♡

Now, if you like, you can write down your current weight. Whatever the result is, don't be too influenced by it.
If it's positive, celebrate!
If not, still be proud of yourself. If you've made it this far, it means you really want to make it.
KEEP STRONG and apply the diary tips.

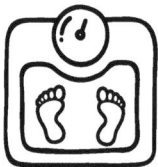

Weight _____

My recommendation is: keep applying the advice of the previous weeks as you strive to take the new little step!

How did the first 7 weeks go?

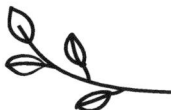

Week 8

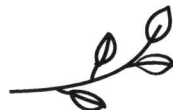

Condiments: Often go unnoticed because they are almost hidden inside our dishes but, in reality, they are one of the main obstacles to weight loss.
By paying attention to which condiments you use and how you dose them you can have benefits on your figure and on your health in a very short time. Let's see the main groups into which the condiments can be divided:

Vegetable oils	Extra Virgin Olive, Seed Oil (Peanuts, Linen, Sesame, Sunflower, ...)
Vinegars and Citrus Juices	wine vinegar, Apple vinegar, Balsamic, Lemon Juice, Orange Juice
Spices and Aromatic Herbs	Salt, Pepper, Thyme, Oregano, Rosemary, Sage, Turmeric, Curry, ...
Animal fats	Butter, Cream, Lard
Gastronomic sauces	Mayonnaise, Mustard, Gastronomic Glazes, Dressing, ...

YES: Extra Virgin Olive Oil. Rich in unsaturated fats, it can protect your arteries by keeping cholesterol levels at bay. You can use up to 2 tablespoons in each meal (including what you put in for cooking): try not to exceed this amount.
NO: Condiments derived from Animal Fats and Gastronomic Sauces. Being high in saturated fat, they promote weight gain and above all cholesterol levels, exposing you to a greater risk of disease.

We land on **SALT:** I recommend that you immediately reduce the salt you add to your dishes. Try not to put the salt shaker on the table anymore and use only what is necessary for cooking, reducing it to the bare minimum. The main reasons why you should do this are:

- Causes water retention which results in swelling and cellulite
- Increases blood pressure and the risk of cardiovascular disease

❧ Small Step of The Week: ❧
IN AT LEAST THREE DIFFERENT DAYS:
DO NOT USE GASTRONOMIC SAUCES
DO NOT TAKE SALT TO THE TABLE
GIVE IT A TRY!

Day 50

Date ___ / ___ / ___

Breakfast

Lunch

Dinner

Snack 1

Snack 2

- Water
- Sleep
- KCal

What time did you eat? Write B for Breakfast, S1 for Snack 1, S2 for Snack 2, L for Lunch, D for Dinner

5 6 7 8 9 10 11 12 13 14 15 16 17 18 19 20 21 22 23 24+

Physical Activities Minutes / Laps / Sets / ...

- ☐ Fast Walking
- ☐ Running
- ☐ Aerobics / Zumba
- ☐ Yoga / Pilates
- ☐
- ☐

Today's Notes

Drugs & Supplements

Bad Habits

MOOD

Don't wait for your ship to arrive to the harbor, swim towards it.

Day (51)

Date ___ / ___ / ___

Breakfast

_____
_____
_____
_____
_____
_____
_____
_____

Lunch

_____
_____
_____
_____
_____
_____
_____
_____

Dinner

_____
_____
_____
_____
_____
_____
_____

Snack 1

_____
_____
_____

Snack 2

_____
_____
_____

Water _____
Sleep _____
KCal _____

What time did you eat? Write B for Breakfast, S1 for Snack 1, S2 for Snack 2, L for Lunch, D for Dinner

5   6   7   8   9   10   11   12   13   14   15   16   17   18   19   20   21   22   23   24+

Physical Activities Minutes / Laps / Sets / ...

- [ ] Fast Walking
- [ ] Running
- [ ] Aerobics / Zumba
- [ ] Yoga / Pilates
- [ ]
- [ ]

Today's Notes

_____
_____

Drugs & Supplements

Bad Habits

MOOD

Day (52)

Date _____ / ____ / ____

Breakfast

Lunch

Dinner

_____
_____
_____
_____
_____
_____
_____

Snack 1

Snack 2

_____
_____
_____
_____

Water _____

Sleep _____

KCal _____

What time did you eat? Write B for Breakfast, S1 for Snack 1, S2 for Snack 2, L for Lunch, D for Dinner

5   6   7   8   9   10   11   12   13   14   15   16   17   18   19   20   21   22   23   24+

Physical Activities   Minutes / Laps / Sets / ...

☐ Fast Walking _____
☐ Running _____
☐ Aerobics / Zumba _____
☐ Yoga / Pilates _____
☐ _____
☐ _____

Today's Notes

Drugs & Supplements

_____
_____
_____
_____

Bad Habits

MOOD

😟   😐   😊

Day 53

Date _____ / _____ / _____

Breakfast

_____
_____
_____
_____
_____
_____
_____

Lunch

_____
_____
_____
_____
_____
_____
_____

Dinner

_____
_____
_____
_____
_____
_____
_____

Snack 1

_____
_____
_____

Snack 2

_____
_____
_____

Water _____
Sleep _____
KCal _____

What time did you eat? Write B for Breakfast, S1 for Snack 1, S2 for Snack 2, L for Lunch, D for Dinner

5   6   7   8   9   10   11   12   13   14   15   16   17   18   19   20   21   22   23   24+

Physical Activities   Minutes / Laps / Sets / ...

☐ Fast Walking   _____
☐ Running   _____
☐ Aerobics / Zumba   _____
☐ Yoga / Pilates   _____
☐   _____
☐   _____

Today's Notes

Drugs & Supplements

Bad Habits

MOOD

Day 54

Date ___ / ___ / ___

Breakfast	Lunch	Dinner

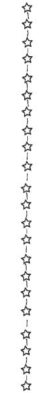 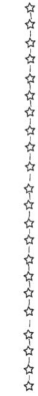

Snack 1	Snack 2	

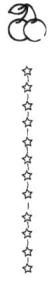 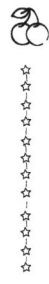

Water ___

Sleep ___

KCal ___

What time did you eat? Write B for Breakfast, S1 for Snack 1, S2 for Snack 2, L for Lunch, D for Dinner

5   6   7   8   9   10   11   12   13   14   15   16   17   18   19   20   21   22   23   24+

♥ Physical Activities   Minutes / Laps / Sets / ...

- ☐ Fast Walking
- ☐ Running
- ☐ Aerobics / Zumba
- ☐ Yoga / Pilates
- ☐
- ☐

🍃 Today's Notes

Drugs & Supplements

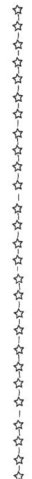

🚭 Bad Habits

MOOD

Day 55

Date ___/___/___

Breakfast
_____
_____
_____
_____
_____
_____
_____

Lunch
_____
_____
_____
_____
_____
_____
_____

Dinner
_____
_____
_____
_____
_____
_____
_____

Snack 1
_____
_____
_____

Snack 2
_____
_____
_____

Water _____
Sleep _____
KCal _____

What time did you eat? Write B for Breakfast, S1 for Snack 1, S2 for Snack 2, L for Lunch, D for Dinner

5 6 7 8 9 10 11 12 13 14 15 16 17 18 19 20 21 22 23 24+

Physical Activities Minutes / Laps / Sets / ...

- [ ] Fast Walking _____
- [ ] Running _____
- [ ] Aerobics / Zumba _____
- [ ] Yoga / Pilates _____
- [ ] _____
- [ ] _____

Today's Notes
_____
_____
_____

Drugs & Supplements
_____
_____
_____
_____

Bad Habits

MOOD
😦 😐 😊

Remain focused on your goals and you won't even notice the obstacles you'll overcome while reaching them

Day 56

Date ___ / ___ / ___

Breakfast

....
....
....
....
....
....

Lunch

....
....
....
....
....
....

Dinner

....
....
....
....
....
....

Snack 1

....
....
....

Snack 2

....
....
....

Water _____

Sleep _____

KCal _____

What time did you eat? Write B for Breakfast, S1 for Snack 1, S2 for Snack 2, L for Lunch, D for Dinner

5   6   7   8   9   10   11   12   13   14   15   16   17   18   19   20   21   22   23   24+

Physical Activities Minutes / Laps / Sets / ...

☐ Fast Walking
☐ Running
☐ Aerobics / Zumba
☐ Yoga / Pilates
☐
☐

Today's Notes

Drugs & Supplements

Bad Habits

MOOD

Eighth Week Check Point

Review what you wrote this week and answer the questions:

1) How many times have you avoided putting the salt cellar on the table?

2) How many times have you avoided putting Gastronomic Sauces on the table?

3) How many times have you used only 2 tablespoons of oil in each meal?

4) Have you experimented with using any spices or aromatic herbs instead of salt?

If you answered at least 3 to the first and second questions you have reached this week's goal and can mark a nice "X" on the Week 8 star. If you answered "YES" to the third and fourth question, then you went beyond the target, very good! If you didn't do it, don't worry, try to understand what prevented you from doing it and we'll try again next week.

♡ ♡ ♡ ♡ ♡ ♡ Do we take measurements? ♡ ♡ ♡ ♡ ♡ ♡

Date _____

Neck _____
Bust _____
Arms _____
Waist _____
Abdomen _____
Hips _____
Thighs _____
Upper Knee _____
Calf _____
Weight _____

How did the first eight weeks go?

_____
_____
_____
_____
_____
_____
_____
_____

Be proud of yourself for every step that you have made a step forward, even if small, is still a step in the right direction

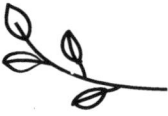

Week 9

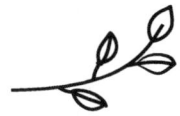

This week we talk about why you should choose "fresh" food over a "packaged" or industrially produced one.

Packaged products, and in particular "snacks", sweets, biscuits, chips, cheese snacks, crackers, breadsticks, wraps, packaged bread, etc. etc., usually contain an excessive amount of sugar, saturated fat, salt and sometimes of chemical additives such as dyes, thickeners and preservatives.

Unfortunately, despite these products being so caloric, they are often also not very "nutritious" and do not satisfy our sense of hunger.

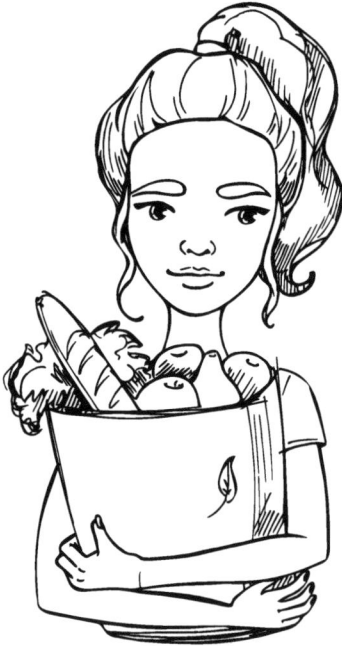

If you are used to consuming packaged products, try replacing them with "fresh" foods and you will immediately see a marked improvement in your physical shape.

You can start by replacing snacks and savory snacks with fruit (fresh or dried). Products purchased fresh can also be frozen without fear of losing their nutritional properties.

If you put packaged bread (or bread sticks) on your table, try replacing it with fresh bread: you can buy it only once a week, cut it into slices and put it in the freezer, this way you can bring out the quantity you need daily.

Small Step Of The Week:

- MAKE 3 SNACKS OR SNACKS USING UNPACKAGED PRODUCTS
- MAKE 3 LUNCHES OR 3 DINNERS USING UNPACKAGED PRODUCTS

GIVE IT A SHOT!

Day 57

Date .... __ / __ / __

Breakfast
_____
_____
_____
_____
_____
_____
_____

Lunch
_____
_____
_____
_____
_____
_____
_____

Dinner
_____
_____
_____
_____
_____
_____
_____

Snack 1
_____
_____
_____

Snack 2
_____
_____
_____

Water _____

Sleep _____

KCal _____

What time did you eat? Write B for Breakfast, S1 for Snack 1, S2 for Snack 2, L for Lunch, D for Dinner

5   6   7   8   9   10   11   12   13   14   15   16   17   18   19   20   21   22   23   24+

Physical Activities   Minutes / Laps / Sets / ...

☐ Fast Walking _____
☐ Running _____
☐ Aerobics / Zumba _____
☐ Yoga / Pilates _____
☐ _____
☐ _____

Today's Notes
_____
_____

Drugs & Supplements
_____
_____
_____
_____

Bad Habits

MOOD
☹ 😐 🙂

Day (58)

Date _____ / ___ / ___

Breakfast

Lunch

Dinner

Snack 1

Snack 2

Water _____

Sleep _____

KCal _____

What time did you eat? Write B for Breakfast, S1 for Snack 1, S2 for Snack 2, L for Lunch, D for Dinner

5   6   7   8   9   10   11   12   13   14   15   16   17   18   19   20   21   22   23   24+

Physical Activities Minutes / Laps / Sets / ...

- ☐ Fast Walking
- ☐ Running
- ☐ Aerobics / Zumba
- ☐ Yoga / Pilates
- ☐
- ☐

Today's Notes

Drugs & Supplements

Bad Habits

MOOD

Don't waste time dwelling on past decisions, focus on future ones.

Day 59

Date ___/___/___

Breakfast

_____
_____
_____
_____
_____
_____

Lunch

_____
_____
_____
_____
_____
_____

Dinner

_____
_____
_____
_____
_____
_____

Snack 1

_____
_____
_____

Snack 2

_____
_____
_____

Water _____

Sleep _____

KCal _____

What time did you eat? Write B for Breakfast, S1 for Snack 1, S2 for Snack 2, L for Lunch, D for Dinner

5   6   7   8   9   10   11   12   13   14   15   16   17   18   19   20   21   22   23   24+

Physical Activities   Minutes / Laps / Sets / ...

☐ Fast Walking _____
☐ Running _____
☐ Aerobics / Zumba _____
☐ Yoga / Pilates _____
☐ _____
☐ _____

Drugs & Supplements

_____
_____
_____
_____

Bad Habits

Today's Notes

_____
_____
_____

MOOD

If you feel like you didn't do enough, be glad. You still did more than nothing.

Day 60

Date ___ / ___ / ___

Breakfast

_____
_____
_____
_____
_____
_____

Lunch

_____
_____
_____
_____
_____
_____

Dinner

_____
_____
_____
_____
_____
_____

Snack 1

_____
_____
_____

Snack 2

_____
_____
_____

Water _____

Sleep _____

KCal _____

What time did you eat? Write B for Breakfast, S1 for Snack 1, S2 for Snack 2, L for Lunch, D for Dinner

5   6   7   8   9   10   11   12   13   14   15   16   17   18   19   20   21   22   23   24+

Physical Activities Minutes / Laps / Sets / ...

- ☐ Fast Walking _____
- ☐ Running _____
- ☐ Aerobics / Zumba _____
- ☐ Yoga / Pilates _____
- ☐ _____
- ☐ _____

Today's Notes

_____
_____
_____

Drugs & Supplements

_____
_____
_____
_____

Bad Habits

MOOD

😟 😐 😊

Stop for a moment and look at how far you've come, all of the efforts were worth it.

Day 61

Date .... __ / __ / __

Breakfast

_____
_____
_____
_____
_____
_____

Lunch

_____
_____
_____
_____
_____
_____

Dinner

_____
_____
_____
_____
_____
_____

Snack 1

_____
_____
_____

Snack 2

_____
_____
_____

Water _____

Sleep _____

KCal _____

What time did you eat? Write B for Breakfast, S1 for Snack 1, S2 for Snack 2, L for Lunch, D for Dinner

5   6   7   8   9   10   11   12   13   14   15   16   17   18   19   20   21   22   23   24+

Physical Activities Minutes / Laps / Sets / ...

- [ ] Fast Walking _____
- [ ] Running _____
- [ ] Aerobics / Zumba _____
- [ ] Yoga / Pilates _____
- [ ] _____
- [ ] _____

Today's Notes

_____
_____

Drugs & Supplements

_____
_____
_____

Bad Habits

MOOD

Day 62

Date ___ / ___ / ___

Breakfast
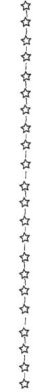
....
....
....
....
....

Lunch
....
....
....
....
....
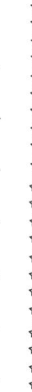

Dinner
....
....
....
....
....

Snack 1
....
....
....

Snack 2
....
....
....

Water ....

Sleep ....

KCal ....

What time did you eat? Write B for Breakfast, S1 for Snack 1, S2 for Snack 2, L for Lunch, D for Dinner

5   6   7   8   9   10   11   12   13   14   15   16   17   18   19   20   21   22   23   24+

Physical Activities Minutes / Laps / Sets / ...

- ☐ Fast Walking ....
- ☐ Running ....
- ☐ Aerobics / Zumba ....
- ☐ Yoga / Pilates ....
- ☐ ....
- ☐ ....

Today's Notes
....
....
....

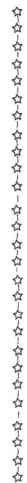

Drugs & Supplements
....
....
....

Bad Habits

MOOD
😕   😐   🙂

Knowing is not enough; we must apply. Willing is not enough; we must do. (Goethe)

Day 63

Date ____ / ____ / ____

Breakfast

Lunch

Dinner

Snack 1

Snack 2

Water _____

Sleep _____

KCal _____

What time did you eat? Write B for Breakfast, S1 for Snack 1, S2 for Snack 2, L for Lunch, D for Dinner

| 5 | 6 | 7 | 8 | 9 | 10 | 11 | 12 | 13 | 14 | 15 | 16 | 17 | 18 | 19 | 20 | 21 | 22 | 23 | 24+ |

Physical Activities
Minutes / Laps / Sets / ...

- [ ] Fast Walking
- [ ] Running
- [ ] Aerobics / Zumba
- [ ] Yoga / Pilates
- [ ]
- [ ]

Today's Notes

Drugs & Supplements

Bad Habits

MOOD

Ninth Week Check Point

Review what you wrote this week and answer the questions:

1) How many times have you had a snack or snack with non-packaged products?

2) How many times have you had a snack or snack with non-packaged products?

If you answered at least 3 to the first and second questions you have reached this week's goal and can mark a nice "X" on the Week 9 star.
If you didn't do it, don't worry, try to understand what prevented you from doing it and we'll try again next week.

By getting into the habit of using fresh products instead of packaged ones, you will do something useful for your well-being and also for the environment. In fact, you will save all the plastic produced for the packaging of packaged products.

♥ ♥ ♥ ♥ ♥ ♥

Now, if you like, you can write down your current weight. Whatever the result is, don't be too influenced by it.
If it's positive, celebrate!
If not, still be proud of yourself. If you've made it this far, it means you really want to make it.
KEEP STRONG and apply the diary tips.

Weight _____

Review all the tips and try to apply them in the coming weeks. You will see that the results will not take long! Keep applying the advice from previous weeks as you strive to take the new little step. Fill in your Diary every day and reread the sentences on the right mindset to maintain. A positive attitude will be your winning weapon.

How did the first 9 weeks go?

_____
_____
_____
_____
_____
_____
_____
_____
_____
_____
_____
_____

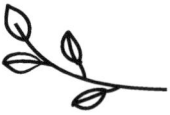

Week 10

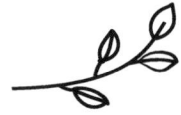

This week's small step will be as easy to do as drinking a glass of water.

We all know how important it is to drink lots of water, but for one reason or another we find ourselves drinking much less than we would need.

Perhaps what not everyone knows is that drinking enough water can also be helpful for limiting weight gain. More often than not, lack of fluids leads us to consume food. This is because dehydration can be confused with a false sense of hunger.

Don't wait until you're thirsty to drink, because thirst comes when you're already dehydrated, rather try to drink at regular intervals.

Moreover, drinking a glass of water before meals can help you reach a sense of satiety earlier.

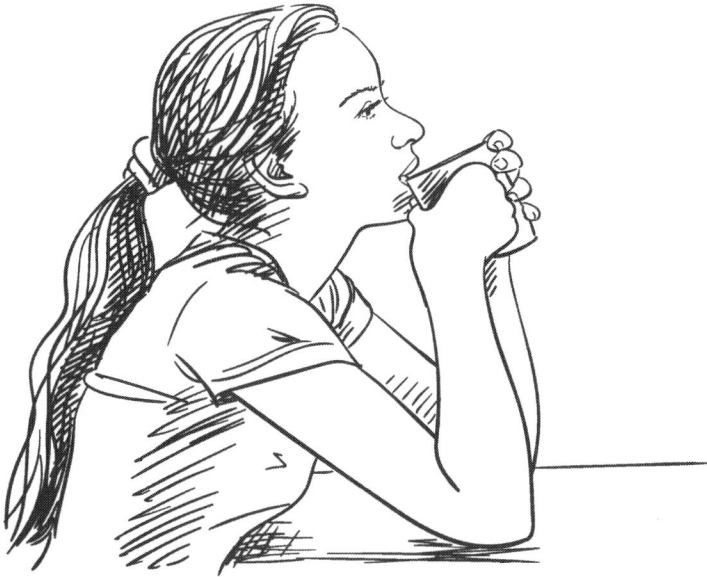

Small Step of the Week:

DRINK AT LEAST ONE AND A HALF LITERS OF WATER A DAY, ON 3 DIFFERENT DAYS.
GIVE IT A TRY!

In your liter and a half count you can also include tea and herbal teas, but the greatest amount must come from water.

Day 64

Date ___ / ___ / ___

Breakfast

....
....
....
....
....
....

Lunch

....
....
....
....
....
....

Dinner

....
....
....
....
....
....

Snack 1

....
....
....
....

Snack 2

....
....
....
....

Water ....

Sleep ....

KCal ....

What time did you eat? Write B for Breakfast, S1 for Snack 1, S2 for Snack 2, L for Lunch, D for Dinner

5   6   7   8   9   10   11   12   13   14   15   16   17   18   19   20   21   22   23   24+

Physical Activities Minutes / Laps / Sets / ...

- ☐ Fast Walking ....
- ☐ Running ....
- ☐ Aerobics / Zumba ....
- ☐ Yoga / Pilates ....
- ☐ ....
- ☐ ....

Drugs & Supplements

....
....
....
....

Bad Habits

Today's Notes

....
....
....
....
....

MOOD

He who has begun has the work half done. (Horace)

Day 65

Date ____ / ____ / ____

Breakfast

_____
_____
_____
_____
_____
_____

Lunch

_____
_____
_____
_____
_____
_____

Dinner

_____
_____
_____
_____
_____
_____

Snack 1

_____
_____
_____

Snack 2

_____
_____
_____

Water _____

Sleep _____

KCal _____

What time did you eat? Write B for Breakfast, S1 for Snack 1, S2 for Snack 2, L for Lunch, D for Dinner

5   6   7   8   9   10   11   12   13   14   15   16   17   18   19   20   21   22   23   24+

Physical Activities   Minutes / Laps / Sets / ...

- ☐ Fast Walking
- ☐ Running
- ☐ Aerobics / Zumba
- ☐ Yoga / Pilates
- ☐
- ☐

Today's Notes

_____
_____
_____

Drugs & Supplements

Bad Habits

MOOD

😕   😐   🙂

If you want to be successful, find someone who has achieved the results you want and copy what they do and you'll achieve the same results. (A. Robbins)

Day 66

Date ___/___/___

Breakfast

Lunch

Dinner

Snack 1

Snack 2

Water _____

Sleep _____

KCal _____

What time did you eat? Write B for Breakfast, S1 for Snack 1, S2 for Snack 2, L for Lunch, D for Dinner

5 6 7 8 9 10 11 12 13 14 15 16 17 18 19 20 21 22 23 24+

Physical Activities Minutes / Laps / Sets / ...

- ☐ Fast Walking
- ☐ Running
- ☐ Aerobics / Zumba
- ☐ Yoga / Pilates
- ☐
- ☐

Today's Notes

Drugs & Supplements

Bad Habits

MOOD

Day 67

Date .... ___ / ___ / ___

Breakfast

Lunch

Dinner

Snack 1

Snack 2

Water _____

Sleep _____

KCal _____

What time did you eat? Write B for Breakfast, S1 for Snack 1, S2 for Snack 2, L for Lunch, D for Dinner

5   6   7   8   9   10   11   12   13   14   15   16   17   18   19   20   21   22   23   24+

Physical Activities   Minutes / Laps / Sets / ...

- [ ] Fast Walking
- [ ] Running
- [ ] Aerobics / Zumba
- [ ] Yoga / Pilates
- [ ]
- [ ]

Drugs & Supplements

Bad Habits

Today's Notes

MOOD

Day 68

Date ____ / ____ / ____

Breakfast

....
....
....
....
....
....

Lunch

....
....
....
....
....
....

Dinner

....
....
....
....
....
....

Snack 1

....
....
....

Snack 2

....
....
....

Water _____
Sleep _____
KCal _____

What time did you eat? Write B for Breakfast, S1 for Snack 1, S2 for Snack 2, L for Lunch, D for Dinner

5   6   7   8   9   10   11   12   13   14   15   16   17   18   19   20   21   22   23   24+

Physical Activities Minutes / Laps / Sets / ...

☐ Fast Walking ....
☐ Running ....
☐ Aerobics / Zumba ....
☐ Yoga / Pilates ....
☐ ....
☐ ....

Today's Notes

Drugs & Supplements

Bad Habits

MOOD

There is only one type of success: doing what you desire with your life. (D. Thoreau)

Day 69

Date ___ / ___ / ___

Breakfast

_____
_____
_____
_____
_____
_____
_____

Lunch

_____
_____
_____
_____
_____
_____
_____

Dinner

_____
_____
_____
_____
_____
_____
_____

Snack 1

_____
_____
_____

Snack 2

_____
_____
_____

Water _____

Sleep _____

KCal _____

What time did you eat? Write B for Breakfast, S1 for Snack 1, S2 for Snack 2, L for Lunch, D for Dinner

5   6   7   8   9   10   11   12   13   14   15   16   17   18   19   20   21   22   23   24+

Physical Activities   Minutes / Laps / Sets / ...

- ☐ Fast Walking
- ☐ Running
- ☐ Aerobics / Zumba
- ☐ Yoga / Pilates
- ☐
- ☐

Today's Notes

_____
_____

Drugs & Supplements

Bad Habits

MOOD

Day 70

Date ___ / ___ / ___

Breakfast

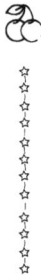

Lunch

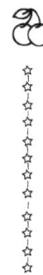

Dinner

Snack 1

Snack 2

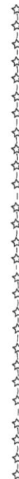

Water _____

Sleep _____

KCal _____

What time did you eat? Write B for Breakfast, S1 for Snack 1, S2 for Snack 2, L for Lunch, D for Dinner

5   6   7   8   9   10   11   12   13   14   15   16   17   18   19   20   21   22   23   24+

Physical Activities   Minutes / Laps / Sets / ...

- ☐ Fast Walking ....
- ☐ Running ....
- ☐ Aerobics / Zumba ....
- ☐ Yoga / Pilates ....
- ☐ ....
- ☐ ....

Today's Notes

Drugs & Supplements

Bad Habits

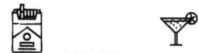
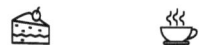

MOOD

☹   😐   🙂

If you're willing to take the chance, the view from the other side is spectacular. (S. Rhimes)

Tenth Week Check Point:

Review what you wrote this week and answer the questions:

1) How many days have you drunk at least one and a half liters of water?

2) How many times have you drunk water even if you were not thirsty?

3) How many times have you tried to drink a glass of water BEFORE meals?

If you answered at least 3 to the first question you have reached this week's goal and can mark a nice "X" on the Week 10 Star.
If you answered "YES" to the second and third questions, then you went beyond the target, very good!
If you didn't do it, don't worry, try to understand what prevented you from doing it and we'll try again next week.

Do not underestimate the importance of drinking enough, water shortage often causes drowsiness, difficulty concentrating and makes us feel in a bad mood, compromising the course of the whole day.

Now, if you like, you can write down your current weight. Don't worry too much if you haven't reached the weight that you thought you should have reached. If you keep working, you can achieve any result.

Weight _____

How did the first
10 weeks go?

_____
_____
_____
_____
_____
_____
_____
_____
_____
_____

NOTICE
Continue to apply the advice of the past weeks in the next few weeks, until they turn into habits. Fill in your diary every day, always read the 3 sentences about the right mindset to maintain and divide what you eat into 5 meals.

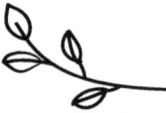

Week 11

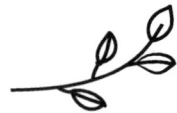

This week we address the topic: "alcoholic and sugary drinks". You may not know that these types of drinks are real enemies for your fitness. Let's see how many calories alcoholic beverages have:

Alcoholic Beverages:	
One glass of Beer	about 100 Kcal
One glass of White Wine	about 110 Kcal
One glass of Red Wine	about 120 Kcal
One glass of Sparkling wine	about 150 Kcal
One Rum & Coke	about 155 Kcal
One Mojito	about 200 Kcal

Doing a simple calculation, if for example we drink a glass of red wine every day for lunch and dinner, we will have added **1680 KCal in a week!** That is the equivalent of 5 full meals, from breakfast to dinner, including snacks!

Sugary Drinks:	
One glass of orangeade	about 135 Kcal
One glass of Coke	about 125 Kcal
One glass of Soda	about 150 Kcal
One non-alcoholic Aperitif	about 150 Kcal
One glass of cold Tea	about 90 Kcal
One glass of Fruit juice	from 135 to 150 Kcal

It seems incredible but to burn off the calories of a single glass of Iced Tea you need to walk 30 minutes! Try to avoid consuming alcohol or sugary drinks every day: **the result will be visible on your weight in a few weeks**

Small Step of The week:

IN AT LEAST 4 DIFFERENT DAYS
DO NOT DRINK ALCOHOLIC OR SUGARED DRINKS
GIVE IT A SHOT!

Day 71

Date ___ / ___ / ___

Breakfast

Lunch

Dinner

Snack 1

Snack 2

🥤 Water _____

🕐 Sleep _____

🍽 KCal _____

What time did you eat? Write B for Breakfast, S1 for Snack 1, S2 for Snack 2, L for Lunch, D for Dinner

5	6	7	8	9	10	11	12	13	14	15	16	17	18	19	20	21	22	23	24+

💓 Physical Activities Minutes / Laps / Sets / ...

- [ ] Fast Walking
- [ ] Running
- [ ] Aerobics / Zumba
- [ ] Yoga / Pilates
- [ ]
- [ ]

🍃 Today's Notes

💊 Drugs & Supplements

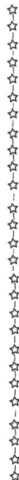

🚭 Bad Habits

MOOD

😟 😐 😊

Day (72)

Date _____ / _____ / _____

Breakfast

....
....
....
....
....
....

Lunch

....
....
....
....
....
....

Dinner

....
....
....
....
....
....

Snack 1

....
....
....

Snack 2

....
....
....

Water

Sleep

KCal

What time did you eat? Write B for Breakfast, S1 for Snack 1, S2 for Snack 2, L for Lunch, D for Dinner

5   6   7   8   9   10   11   12   13   14   15   16   17   18   19   20   21   22   23   24+

Physical Activities Minutes / Laps / Sets / ...

☐ Fast Walking ....
☐ Running ....
☐ Aerobics / Zumba ....
☐ Yoga / Pilates ....
☐ ....
☐ ....

Today's Notes

Drugs & Supplements

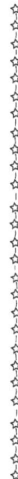

....
....
....
....

Bad Habits

MOOD

Day 73

Date ___ / ___ / ___

Breakfast

_____
_____
_____
_____
_____
_____

Lunch

_____
_____
_____
_____
_____
_____

Dinner

_____
_____
_____
_____
_____
_____

Snack 1

_____
_____
_____

Snack 2

_____
_____
_____

Water _____

Sleep _____

KCal _____

What time did you eat? Write B for Breakfast, S1 for Snack 1, S2 for Snack 2, L for Lunch, D for Dinner

5   6   7   8   9   10   11   12   13   14   15   16   17   18   19   20   21   22   23   24+

Physical Activities Minutes / Laps / Sets / ...

- [ ] Fast Walking   _____
- [ ] Running   _____
- [ ] Aerobics / Zumba   _____
- [ ] Yoga / Pilates   _____
- [ ]   _____
- [ ]   _____

Drugs & Supplements

_____
_____
_____

Bad Habits

Today's Notes

_____
_____

MOOD

Day (74)   Date _____ / ___ / ___

Breakfast   ## Lunch   ## Dinner

_____   _____   _____
_____   _____   _____
_____   _____   _____
_____   _____   _____
_____   _____   _____

Snack 1   ## Snack 2

_____   _____   Water _____
_____   _____   Sleep _____
_____   _____   KCal _____

What time did you eat? Write B for Breakfast, S1 for Snack 1, S2 for Snack 2, L for Lunch, D for Dinner

5 6 7 8 9 10 11 12 13 14 15 16 17 18 19 20 21 22 23 24+

Physical Activities Minutes / Laps / Sets / ...

☐ Fast Walking   _____
☐ Running   _____
☐ Aerobics / Zumba _____
☐ Yoga / Pilates _____
☐   _____
☐   _____

Today's Notes

Drugs & Supplements

_____
_____
_____

Bad Habits

MOOD

Day 75

Date _____ / _____ / _____

Breakfast
_____
_____
_____
_____
_____
_____
_____

Lunch
_____
_____
_____
_____
_____
_____
_____

Dinner
_____
_____
_____
_____
_____
_____
_____

Snack 1
_____
_____
_____

Snack 2
_____
_____
_____

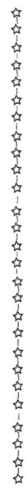

Water
Sleep
KCal

What time did you eat? Write B for Breakfast, S1 for Snack 1, S2 for Snack 2, L for Lunch, D for Dinner

5   6   7   8   9   10   11   12   13   14   15   16   17   18   19   20   21   22   23   24+

💓 Physical Activities   Minutes / Laps / Sets / ...

- ☐ Fast Walking
- ☐ Running
- ☐ Aerobics / Zumba
- ☐ Yoga / Pilates
- ☐
- ☐

🌿 Today's Notes
_____
_____
_____

Drugs & Supplements
_____
_____
_____
_____

Bad Habits

MOOD
☹️   😐   🙂

Look ahead, stay positive and do all you can. Doing this means you have already won!
(J. Rohn)

Day 76

Date ___ / ___ / ___

Breakfast

....
....
....
....
....
....
....
....

Lunch

....
....
....
....
....
....
....
....

Dinner

....
....
....
....
....
....
....
....

Snack 1

....
....
....
....

Snack 2

....
....
....
....

- Water
- Sleep
- KCal

What time did you eat? Write B for Breakfast, S1 for Snack 1, S2 for Snack 2, L for Lunch, D for Dinner

5   6   7   8   9   10   11   12   13   14   15   16   17   18   19   20   21   22   23   24+

Physical Activities Minutes / Laps / Sets / ...

- ☐ Fast Walking ....
- ☐ Running ....
- ☐ Aerobics / Zumba ....
- ☐ Yoga / Pilates ....
- ☐ ....
- ☐ ....

Today's Notes

Drugs & Supplements

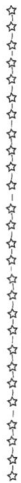

....
....
....
....

Bad Habits

MOOD

Day 77

Date ___ / ___ / ___

Breakfast

_____
_____
_____
_____
_____
_____

Lunch

_____
_____
_____
_____
_____
_____

Dinner

_____
_____
_____
_____
_____
_____

Snack 1

_____
_____
_____

Snack 2

_____
_____
_____

Water _____

Sleep _____

KCal _____

What time did you eat? Write B for Breakfast, S1 for Snack 1, S2 for Snack 2, L for Lunch, D for Dinner

5   6   7   8   9   10   11   12   13   14   15   16   17   18   19   20   21   22   23   24+

Physical Activities Minutes / Laps / Sets / ...

☐ Fast Walking _____
☐ Running _____
☐ Aerobics / Zumba _____
☐ Yoga / Pilates _____
☐ _____
☐ _____

Today's Notes

_____
_____
_____

Drugs & Supplements

_____
_____
_____
_____

Bad Habits

MOOD

Eleventh Week Check Point

Review what you wrote this week and answer the questions:

1) How many times have you drank alcoholic beverages this week?

2) How many times have you drank sugary drinks this week?

If you answered at least 3 to the first and second questions you have reached this week's goal and can mark a nice "X" on the Week 11 star. If you didn't do it, don't worry, try to understand what prevented you from doing it and we'll try again next week.

Do you know that some beliefs about alcoholic beverages are completely unfounded?
For example, it is not true that "beer quenches thirst", on the contrary, the alcohol contained within it causes dehydration because our body will have to use a large amount of water to metabolize it, thus it also stimulates diuresis causing further loss of fluids.
It is not true that "herbal bitters make you digest", on the contrary, due to the alcohol contained within them, they slow down the digestive processes and cause inflammation in the digestive system.

♥ ♥ ♥ ♥ ♥ ♥

How did the first 11 weeks go?

Now if you like, you can write down your current weight if. Whatever the result is, don't be too influenced by it. **If it's positive, celebrate!**

If not, don't lose motivation, the situation is only momentary. Hang in there, stick to your diet, apply the Diary's advice, and you'll soon see the results.

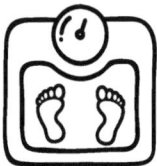

Weight _____

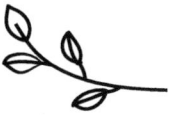

Week 12

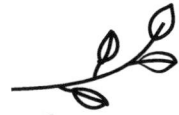

If you also happen to not have the right ingredients for your meals, this week I have some tips that could help you shop and always have what you need.

Getting started: Plan your week in advance.

Draw a table for next week on a slate or a piece of paper and mark the meals you think you should prepare at home with an "X". Once you know how many meals you will need to prepare, you can make a list of everything you need.

	MON	TUE	WED	THU	FRI	SAT	SUN	Total
Breakfast	X	X	X	X	X	X		6
Snack 1	X	X	X	X	X	X		6
Lunch	X		X		X	X	X	5
Snack 2	X	X	X	X	X			5
Dinner		X		X			X	3

In this example I planned to have to prepare at home:

6 Breakfasts,
6 Snacks 1,
5 Lunches,
5 Snacks 2,
3 Dinners.

On the side I bring you the shopping list that I put together based on the meals provided in the table above.

Fresh and frozen Vegetables	Salad x 8 meals (lunches and dinners) 5 Lunches: 2 times zucchini, 1 time eggplants, 2 times tomatoes 3 Dinners: 1 time spinach, one time beets, one time artichokes. Some Celery and Carrots for the Snacks
Fresh Fruit	6 fruits for Snack 1 5 fruits for Lunch 3 fruits for Dinner
Dried Fruit	6 servings of walnuts for Snack
Pasta / Grain Cereals / Potatoes	4 Lunches: 1 Wholemeal Pasta, 1 Rice, 1 Quinoa, 1 Couscous 3 Dinners: 2 times bread, 1 time potatoes
Bread	Wholemeal bread for 2 dinners (one doesn't need because I have potatoes)
Breakfast Cereals	6 breakfasts: Muesli x 5 breakfasts + Wholemeal biscuits for the sixth breakfast
Fish	Mackerel Monday lunch + Shrimps Wed lunch+ Bream for Saturday Lunch Cod for Tuesday Dinner
White Meat	Chicken for Friday's Lunch + Turkey for Sunday's Lunch
Red Meat	Beef for Tuesday's dinner
Processed Meats	This week nothing, Next Week I'll buy ham
Legumes	Lentils for 1 Tuesday's dinner, Minestrone soup for one lunch
Dairy products	Milk for 6 breakfasts + Feta for the Couscous
Eggs	2 eggs for Thursday's dinner+ 2 for Sunday's breakfast pancake

Small Step of The week:

PLAN YOUR WEEK IN ADVANCE. GIVE IT A TRY!

Day 78

Date ___ / ___ / ___

Breakfast

Lunch

Dinner

Snack 1

Snack 2

🥛 Water ___
⏰ Sleep ___
🍽 KCal ___

What time did you eat? Write B for Breakfast, S1 for Snack 1, S2 for Snack 2, L for Lunch, D for Dinner

5   6   7   8   9   10   11   12   13   14   15   16   17   18   19   20   21   22   23   24+

Physical Activities Minutes / Laps / Sets / ...

- ☐ Fast Walking
- ☐ Running
- ☐ Aerobics / Zumba
- ☐ Yoga / Pilates
- ☐
- ☐

Today's Notes

Drugs & Supplements

Bad Habits

MOOD

Chase your dreams, don't give up in front of anything. Make your life spectacular.

Day (79)

Date ___ / ___ / ___

Breakfast

_____
_____
_____
_____
_____
_____

Lunch

_____
_____
_____
_____
_____
_____

Dinner

_____
_____
_____
_____
_____

Snack 1

_____
_____
_____

Snack 2

_____
_____
_____

Water _____

Sleep _____

KCal _____

What time did you eat? Write B for Breakfast, S1 for Snack 1, S2 for Snack 2, L for Lunch, D for Dinner

5   6   7   8   9   10   11   12   13   14   15   16   17   18   19   20   21   22   23   24+

Physical Activities   Minutes / Laps / Sets / ...

☐ Fast Walking _____
☐ Running _____
☐ Aerobics / Zumba _____
☐ Yoga / Pilates _____
☐ _____
☐ _____

Drugs & Supplements

Today's Notes

_____
_____

Bad Habits

MOOD

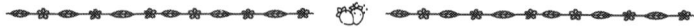

Day 80

Date ____ / ____ / ____

Breakfast

_____
_____
_____
_____
_____
_____

Lunch

_____
_____
_____
_____
_____
_____

Dinner

_____
_____
_____
_____
_____
_____

Snack 1

_____
_____
_____

Snack 2

_____
_____
_____

Water _____
Sleep _____
KCal _____

What time did you eat? Write B for Breakfast, S1 for Snack 1, S2 for Snack 2, L for Lunch, D for Dinner

5   6   7   8   9   10   11   12   13   14   15   16   17   18   19   20   21   22   23   24+

Physical Activities Minutes / Laps / Sets / ...

☐ Fast Walking ....
☐ Running ....
☐ Aerobics / Zumba ....
☐ Yoga / Pilates ....
☐ ....
☐ ....

Today's Notes

_____
_____
_____
_____

Drugs & Supplements

Bad Habits

MOOD

In life there are only two rules: 1) Never give up; 2) Never forget rule number 1.

Day (81)   Date ___ / ___ / ___

Breakfast
_____
_____
_____
_____
_____
_____

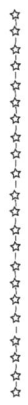

Lunch
_____
_____
_____
_____
_____
_____

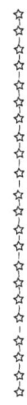

Dinner
_____
_____
_____
_____
_____
_____

Snack 1
_____
_____
_____

Snack 2
_____
_____
_____

Water _____
Sleep _____
KCal _____

What time did you eat? Write B for Breakfast, S1 for Snack 1, S2 for Snack 2, L for Lunch, D for Dinner

5   6   7   8   9   10   11   12   13   14   15   16   17   18   19   20   21   22   23   24+

Physical Activities   Minutes / Laps / Sets / ...

☐ Fast Walking _____
☐ Running _____
☐ Aerobics / Zumba _____
☐ Yoga / Pilates _____
☐ _____
☐ _____

Today's Notes
_____
_____

Drugs & Supplements
_____
_____
_____
_____

Bad Habits

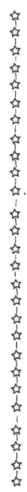

MOOD
☹   😐   😊

Above all, don't fear difficult moments. The best comes from them. (Rita Levi-Montalcini)

Day (82)

Date ____ / ____ / ____

Breakfast

....
....
....
....
....
....
....

Lunch

....
....
....
....
....
....
....

Dinner

....
....
....
....
....
....
....

Snack 1

....
....
....

Snack 2

....
....
....

Water ....

Sleep ....

KCal ....

What time did you eat? Write B for Breakfast, S1 for Snack 1, S2 for Snack 2, L for Lunch, D for Dinner

5	6	7	8	9	10	11	12	13	14	15	16	17	18	19	20	21	22	23	24+

Physical Activities Minutes / Laps / Sets / ...

- [ ] Fast Walking ....
- [ ] Running ....
- [ ] Aerobics / Zumba ....
- [ ] Yoga / Pilates ....
- [ ] ....
- [ ] ....

Drugs & Supplements

....
....

Bad Habits

Today's Notes

....
....
....

MOOD

Just make sure you never do less than your best. (W. Disney)

Day (83)

Date ____ / ____ / ____

Breakfast

Lunch

Dinner

Snack 1

Snack 2

Water ____

Sleep ____

KCal ____

What time did you eat? Write B for Breakfast, S1 for Snack 1, S2 for Snack 2, L for Lunch, D for Dinner

| 5 | 6 | 7 | 8 | 9 | 10 | 11 | 12 | 13 | 14 | 15 | 16 | 17 | 18 | 19 | 20 | 21 | 22 | 23 | 24+ |

Physical Activities Minutes / Laps / Sets / ...

- [ ] Fast Walking
- [ ] Running
- [ ] Aerobics / Zumba
- [ ] Yoga / Pilates
- [ ]
- [ ]

Drugs & Supplements

Bad Habits

Today's Notes

MOOD

Day (84)

Date ___ / ___ / ___

Breakfast

Lunch

Dinner

Snack 1

Snack 2

Water _____

Sleep _____

KCal _____

What time did you eat? Write B for Breakfast, S1 for Snack 1, S2 for Snack 2, L for Lunch, D for Dinner

5   6   7   8   9   10   11   12   13   14   15   16   17   18   19   20   21   22   23   24+

Physical Activities Minutes / Laps / Sets / ...

☐ Fast Walking

☐ Running

☐ Aerobics / Zumba

☐ Yoga / Pilates

☐

☐

Today's Notes

Drugs & Supplements

Bad Habits

MOOD

Our greatest weakness lies in giving up.
The most certain way to succeed is always to try just one more time. (Thomas Edison)

Twelfth Week Check Point

Review what you wrote this week and answer the questions:

1) Have you tried to plan meals for the whole week in advance? ☐

2) Have you compiled a shopping list taking into account the meals to be prepared? ☐

If you answered "Yes" to the 2 questions you have reached this week's goal and can mark a nice "X" on the Week 12 star. If you didn't do it, don't worry, try to understand what prevented you from doing it and we'll try again next week.

Are you managing to turn all the little steps you have taken into good habits? Try to answer these questions to make a point of the situation:

1) How many times have you done at least 30 minutes of physical activity a day? ☐

2) How many times have you drank at least one and a half liters of water in a day? ☐

3) How many times have you had a healthy and balanced breakfast? ☐

4) How many times have you consumed whole grains instead of refined ones? ☐

5) How many times have you followed the healthy dish rule? ☐

6) How many times have you only had 5 meals at day? ☐

7) How many times have you eaten fresh fruit as a snack? ☐

♡ ♡ ♡ ♡ ♡ ♡

How did this 12 weeks go?

Now if you like, you can write down your current weight if. Whatever the result is, don't be too influenced by it.
If it's positive, celebrate!

If not, don't lose motivation, the situation is only momentary. **Every day can be a new starting point and from tomorrow you can already do better.**

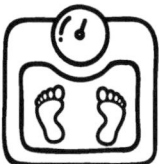

Weight _____

_____

_____

_____

_____

_____

_____

_____

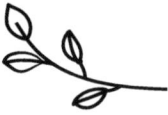

Week 13

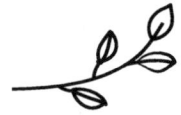

Did you notice how far we traveled to get here?
You have faced many challenges and worked so hard to overcome them, now is the time to think about something that is essential to keep your body and mind healthy: TAKE CARE OF YOURSELF.

Many people neglect this aspect, but it would be really better not to because an excessive load of stress increases the cortisol levels in the blood and this leads, in the long term, to gain weight or not to lose weight even if you follow a diet. It is often said: "If you want to lose weight first Relax", and it's true!

What is the time of day when you feel the most stressed and nervous? Have you noticed if on those occasions you find yourself overeating?

To avoid doing this, look for an outlet that allows you to release your nervousness, such as going out for a run.
Your daily routine needs to be organized so that you can take some time for yourself. If you can't do it during the day, then set aside 15 minutes for relaxation before going to bed.

Whenever you have a bad moment instead of throwing yourself on food, take a deep breath, put on your headphones and listen to your favorite songs for a few minutes.

I assure you it works!

Even flying with your mind can be relaxing, you are already starting to think about the trip you would like to do so much, look for information, write down an itinerary. Having a future goal already planned helps you deal better with the classic work and family routine.

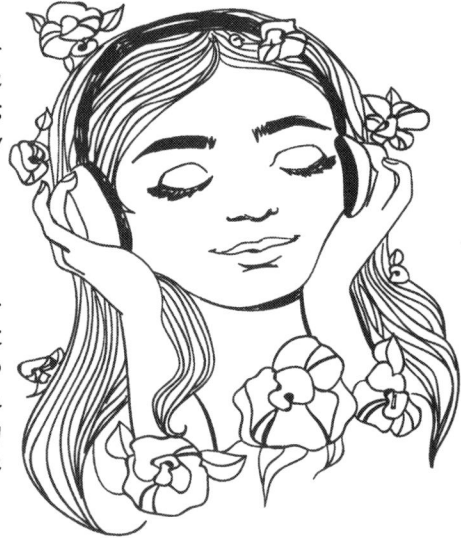

Small Step of the Week:

ORGANIZE SOMETHING FOR YOURSELF, TO DO IN NOT TOO LONG TERM: A WEEKEND OUTSIDE OF TOWN, A DINNER WITH FRIENDS, OR JUST AN AFTERNOON AT THE SPA.

GIVE IT A TRY!

Day 85

Date ___ / ___ / ___

Breakfast

_____
_____
_____
_____
_____
_____
_____

Lunch

_____
_____
_____
_____
_____
_____
_____

Dinner

_____
_____
_____
_____
_____
_____
_____

Snack 1

_____
_____
_____

Snack 2

_____
_____
_____

Water _____

Sleep _____

KCal _____

What time did you eat? Write B for Breakfast, S1 for Snack 1, S2 for Snack 2, L for Lunch, D for Dinner

5 6 7 8 9 10 11 12 13 14 15 16 17 18 19 20 21 22 23 24+

Physical Activities Minutes / Laps / Sets / ...

- [ ] Fast Walking _____
- [ ] Running _____
- [ ] Aerobics / Zumba _____
- [ ] Yoga / Pilates _____
- [ ] _____
- [ ] _____

Today's Notes

_____
_____
_____

Drugs & Supplements

_____
_____
_____

Bad Habits

MOOD

Be proud of everything you've done and everything you are!

Day 86

Date ___ / ___ / ___

Breakfast
....
....
....
....
....
....
....

Lunch
....
....
....
....
....
....
....

Dinner
....
....
....
....
....
....
....

Snack 1
....
....
....

Snack 2
....
....
....

Water ....

Sleep ....

KCal ....

What time did you eat? Write B for Breakfast, S1 for Snack 1, S2 for Snack 2, L for Lunch, D for Dinner

5   6   7   8   9   10   11   12   13   14   15   16   17   18   19   20   21   22   23   24+

Physical Activities   Minutes / Laps / Sets / ...

☐ Fast Walking ....
☐ Running ....
☐ Aerobics / Zumba ....
☐ Yoga / Pilates ....
☐ ....
☐ ....

Today's Notes
....
....
....

Drugs & Supplements
....
....
....
....

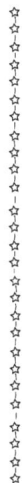

Bad Habits
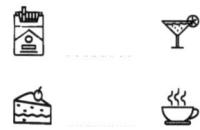

MOOD
:(:| :)

Day 87

Date ___ / ___ / ___

Breakfast

_____
_____
_____
_____
_____
_____

Lunch

_____
_____
_____
_____
_____
_____

Dinner

_____
_____
_____
_____
_____
_____

Snack 1

_____
_____
_____

Snack 2

_____
_____
_____

Water _____

Sleep _____

KCal _____

What time did you eat? Write B for Breakfast, S1 for Snack 1, S2 for Snack 2, L for Lunch, D for Dinner

5   6   7   8   9   10   11   12   13   14   15   16   17   18   19   20   21   22   23   24+

Physical Activities   Minutes / Laps / Sets / ...

☐ Fast Walking _____
☐ Running _____
☐ Aerobics / Zumba _____
☐ Yoga / Pilates _____
☐ _____
☐ _____

Drugs & Supplements

_____
_____
_____

Bad Habits

Today's Notes

_____
_____
_____

MOOD

To reach your goals you have to believe in yourself with your whole heart.

Day 88

Date ___ / ___ / ___

Breakfast

Lunch

Dinner

Snack 1

Snack 2

- Water
- Sleep
- KCal

What time did you eat? Write B for Breakfast, S1 for Snack 1, S2 for Snack 2, L for Lunch, D for Dinner

| 5 | 6 | 7 | 8 | 9 | 10 | 11 | 12 | 13 | 14 | 15 | 16 | 17 | 18 | 19 | 20 | 21 | 22 | 23 | 24+ |

Physical Activities Minutes / Laps / Sets / ...

- ☐ Fast Walking
- ☐ Running
- ☐ Aerobics / Zumba
- ☐ Yoga / Pilates
- ☐
- ☐

Today's Notes

Drugs & Supplements

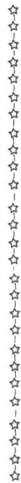

Bad Habits

MOOD

You're almost there! Hold on for a couple more days and you'll see wonderful results.

Day 89

Date ___/___/___

Breakfast	Lunch	Dinner

Snack 1

Snack 2

Water

Sleep

KCal

What time did you eat? Write B for Breakfast, S1 for Snack 1, S2 for Snack 2, L for Lunch, D for Dinner

5   6   7   8   9   10   11   12   13   14   15   16   17   18   19   20   21   22   23   24+

Physical Activities   Minutes / Laps / Sets / ...

- ☐ Fast Walking
- ☐ Running
- ☐ Aerobics / Zumba
- ☐ Yoga / Pilates
- ☐
- ☐

Today's Notes

Drugs & Supplements

Bad Habits

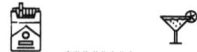

MOOD

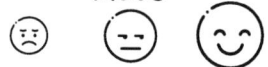

True strength is when you go through difficult moments and decide to not give up.

Day 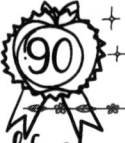 Date ___ / ___ / ___

Breakfast

Lunch

Dinner

_____
_____
_____
_____
_____
_____
_____

Snack 1

Snack 2

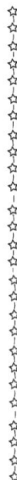

🥛 Water

⏰ Sleep

🍽️ KCal

What time did you eat? Write B for Breakfast, S1 for Snack 1, S2 for Snack 2, L for Lunch, D for Dinner

5　6　7　8　9　10　11　12　13　14　15　16　17　18　19　20　21　22　23　24+

💓 Physical Activities Minutes / Laps / Sets / ...

☐ Fast Walking ....

☐ Running ....

☐ Aerobics / Zumba ....

☐ Yoga / Pilates ....

☐ ....

☐ ....

💊 Drugs & Supplements

🚭 Bad Habits

🚬　🍸

🍰　☕

🍃 Today's Notes

MOOD

😒　😐　😊

Give every day the chance to become the most beautiful day of your life. (M. Twain)

Thirteenth Week Check Point

Review what you wrote this week and answer the questions:

1) Have you planned something to do to take care of yourself?

2) How many times have you managed to take 15 minutes for relaxation?

If you answered "YES" to the first question you have reached this week's goal and can mark a nice "X" on the Week 13 Star. If you answered at least 2 to the second question, then you went beyond the target, very good!

Did you know that sleeping at night also affects the ability to lose weight?
This happens because lack of sleep negatively affects the hormones that regulate hunger and can lead to an increased risk of obesity and diabetes.
To improve your night's rest, you can try not to use tablets, PCs or mobile phones half an hour before going to bed. This will prevent screen lights from adversely affecting natural melatonin production.

♡ ♡ ♡ ♡ ♡ ♡

On the next page you will find the scheme for recording your weight and your measurements and a thought on how to continue your journey. Below I leave you the space to describe how you feel after these 13 weeks with the company of Your Diary.

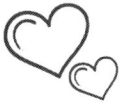

How did this 13
weeks go?

_____

_____

_____

_____

_____

Measurements at day 90

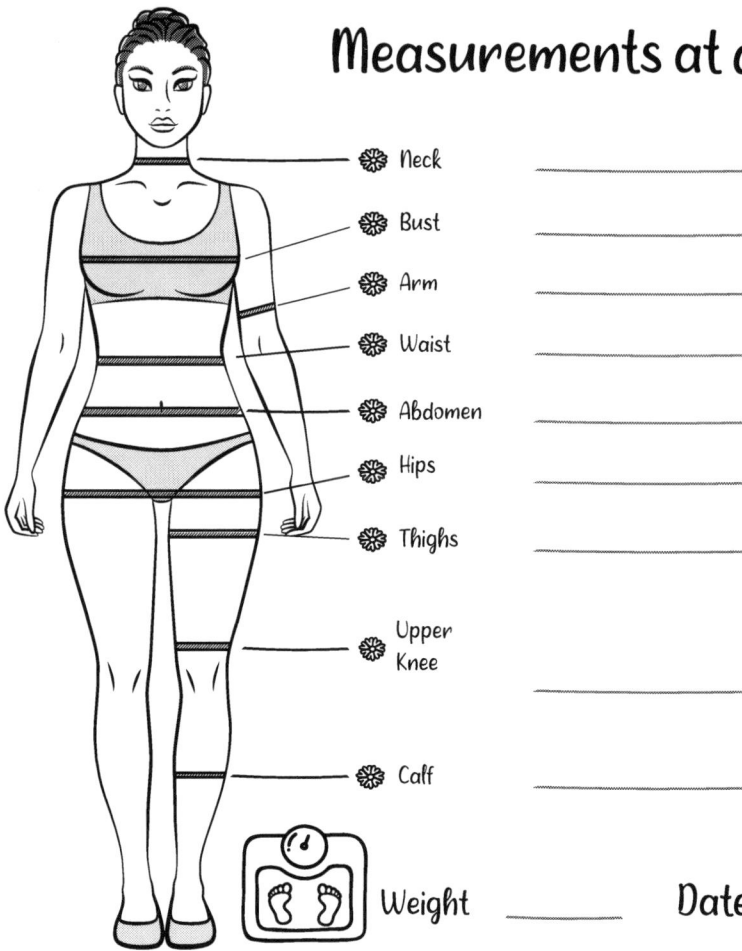

🌸 Neck _____

🌸 Bust _____

🌸 Arm _____

🌸 Waist _____

🌸 Abdomen _____

🌸 Hips _____

🌸 Thighs _____

🌸 Upper
Knee _____

🌸 Calf _____

Weight _____ Date _____

♡ ♡ ♡ ♡ ♡ ♡

How to move forward

First I have to congratulate you, if you have come this far you are a person who does not give up easily.

If you have achieved the goal you set, it means that, thanks to your commitment and determination, you have changed your lifestyle to get what you wanted. Continue like this until all the small steps you have taken become habits so deeply rooted within you that they no longer are an effort.

If you haven't reached your goal yet, you can take the advice from this diary and try again, after all it's only been 90 days! You have all the time you need in front of you.

The road to becoming the best version of yourself must be traveled without any rush to obtain results that last over time. **Enjoy the journey and always be proud of yourself.**

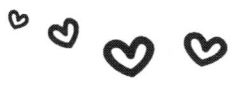
My Thoughts.
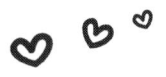

....

....

....

....

....

....

....

....

....

....

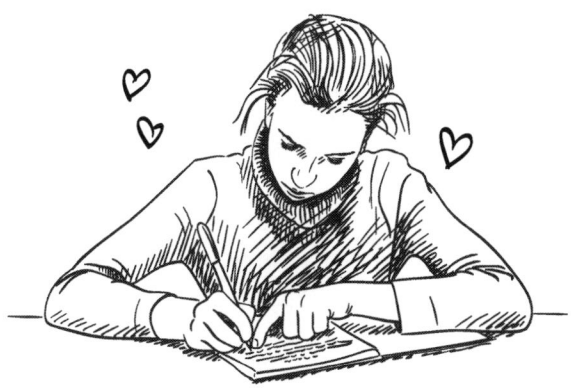

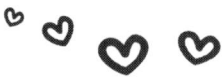# My Thoughts.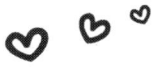

....

....

....

....

....

....

....

....

....

....

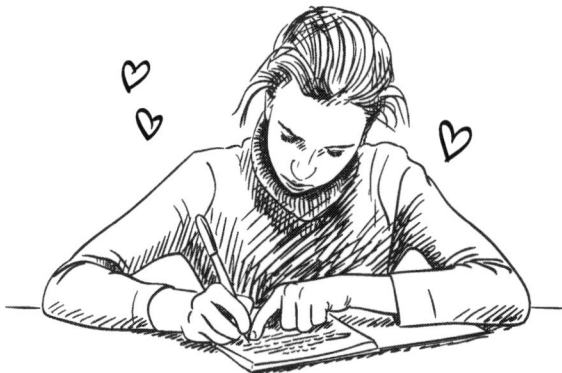

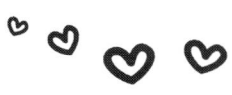

My Thoughts.

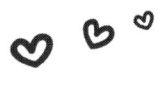

....

....

....

....

....

....

....

....

....

....

....

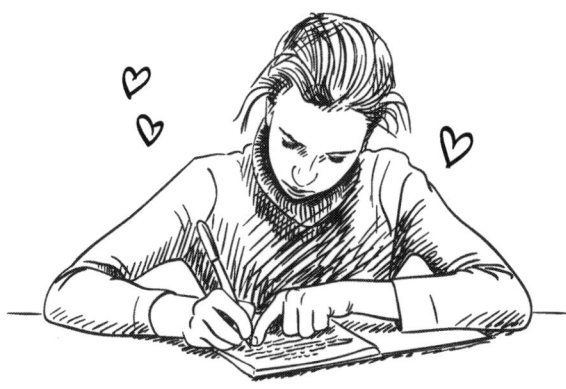

YOUR OPINION MATTERS

This Diary was created by Biologist Nutritionist Dr. Simona Meloni with the aim of being of help to all those who want to improve their eating habits. To find out more about me you can visit my Facebook Profile (facebook.com/Nutritionists.Recipes) or follow my Instagram profile @dssa.simona.nutrizionista.

If you would like to give me some advice on how to improve the next version of this diary or stay up to date on upcoming publications you can email me at:

info@effectspublishing.com

Thank you for your recent purchase. I hope you love it! If you do, would you consider posting a review on Amazon?
This helps me to continue providing great products and helps potential buyers to make confident decisions.

Scientific Resources:
Consiglio per la ricerca in agricoltura e l'analisi dell'economia agraria (CREA)
Harvard T.H. Chan School of Public Health

Sian Porter (British Dietetic Association)

ISBN: 9798594647107 (Paperback - color orange)
ISBN: 9798597724478 (Paperback - color blue)
First printing edition January 2021.

Dr. Simona Meloni, Nutritionist / EffectsPublishing - Email: info@effectspublishing.com

Credits:
All images are fully licensed for commercial use by Shutterstock and Adobe Stock
Some license free icons come from www.flaticon.com
Authors of Icons are Flaticon , Good Ware, Freepik , Dooder. Please let we know if some credits is missing.

Printed in Great Britain
by Amazon

69326539R00078